Quality Management
in Prehospital Care

Quality Management in Prehospital Care

BY THE
NATIONAL ASSOCIATION OF EMS PHYSICIANS

CHIEF EDITOR

ROBERT A. SWOR, D.O., F.A.C.E.P.
EMS Director,
William Beaumont Hospital–Royal Oak
Clinical Instructor, Section of Emergency Medicine,
Department of Surgery, University of Michigan
Royal Oak, Michigan

EDITORS

STEVEN J. ROTTMAN, M.D., F.A.C.E.P.
Professor of Medicine, Division of Emergency Medicine
Director, UCLA Center for Prehospital Care
Medical Director, City of Burbank EMS
Los Angeles, California

RONALD G. PIRRALLO, M.D.
SAEM Physio-Control Fellow in EMS,
Department of Emergency Medicine,
William Beaumont Hospital–Royal Oak
Royal Oak, Michigan

ERIC DAVIS, M.D., F.A.C.E.P.
Assistant Professor of Medicine,
Division of Emergency Medicine, University of Pittsburgh
Medical Director, STAT System
Wexford, Pennsylvania

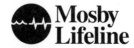

Mosby Lifeline

St. Louis Baltimore Boston Chicago London Philadelphia Sydney Toronto

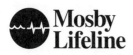

Senior Editor: Claire Merrick
Developmental Editor: Nancy J. Peterson
Assistant Editor: Dana Battaglia
Production Editor: Ross Goldberg

Copyright © 1993 by Mosby–Year Book, Inc.
A Mosby Lifeline imprint of Mosby–Year Book, Inc.

Printed in the United States of America

Mosby–Year Book Inc.
11830 Westline Industrial Drive
St. Louis, Missouri 63146

Library of Congress Cataloging in Publication Data

Quality management in prehospital care / by the National Association
  of EMS Physicians; chief editor, Robert A. Swor; editors, Steven J.
  Rottman, Ronald G. Pirrallo, Eric Davis.
    p.   cm.
  Includes bibliographical references and index.
  ISBN 0-8016-6579-5
  1. Emergency medical services—Quality control. I. Swor, Robert
A. II. National Association of EMS Physicians (U.S.)
  [DNLM: 1. Emergency Medical Services—organization &
administration.   2. Quality Assurance, Health Care—organization &
administration.   WX 215   Q13]
RA645.5.Q36   1993
362.1'8'068—dc20
DNLM/DLC
for Library of Congress   92-49237
                                                                      CIP

92 93 94 95 96 CL/MY 9 8 7 6 5 4 3 2 1

Contents

Contributing Authors

Maria B. Abrahamsen, J.D.
Partner,
Law Offices of Dykema Gossett
Detroit, Michigan

Nicholas Benson, M.D., F.A.C.E.P.
Associate Professor of Emergency
Medicine,
East Carolina School of Medicine
Chairman, EMS Committee,
American College of Emergency
Physicians
Greenville, North Carolina

Garry Briese, CAE
Executive Director,
International Association of Fire Chiefs
Washington, D.C.

Brenda Bruns, M.D., F.A.C.E.P.
EMS Medical Director,
Emergency Medical Service District
Alameda County, California

Kathleen A. Cline, M.D., F.A.C.E.P.
Greenville, North Carolina

Peter A. Curka, D.O., F.A.C.E.P.
Assistant Medical Director for Quality
Assurance and Direct Medical Control,
City of Houston Emergency Medical
Services
Instructor, Department of Medicine,
Baylor College of Medicine
Houston, Texas

Steven J. Davidson, M.D., M.B.A.,
F.A.C.E.P.
Professor of Emergency Medicine and
Division Head,
Division of Emergency Medical Services,
Medical College of Pennsylvania
Medical Director of EMS,
Philadelphia Fire Department
Regional EMS Medical Director,
Philadelphia, Pennsylvania

Eric Davis, M.D., F.A.C.E.P.
Assistant Professor of Medicine,
Division of Emergency Medicine,
University of Pittsburgh
Medical Director, STAT System,
Wexford, Pennsylvania

Jim Dernocoeur, EMT–P
Team Dernocoeur
Grand Rapids, Michigan

Timothy Fleming, M.D., F.A.C.E.P.
New Mexico State EMS Medical
Director
Tesuque, New Mexico

Gene W. Kallsen, M.D., M.P.H.,
F.A.C.E.P.
Chief, Emergency Medicine,
Valley Medical Center
Fresno, California

Alexander Kuehl, M.D., M.P.H.,
F.A.C.S.
Director, Emergency Department at
New York Hospital
New York, New York

Ronald F. Maio, D.O., F.A.C.E.P.
Assistant Professor, Section of
Emergency Medicine,
Department of Surgery,
University of Michigan School of
Medicine
Ann Arbor, Michigan

**Richard M. McDowell, M.D.,
F.A.C.E.P.**
Director, Emergency Department,
Conemaugh Hospital
Johnstown, Pennsylvania

Vincent Mosesso, M.D., F.A.C.E.P.
Assistant Professor of Medicine,
Division of Emergency Medicine,
University of Pittsburgh School of
Medicine
Pittsburgh, Pennsylvania

John New, B.A.
Acting Director, Operations Research &
Systems Analysis,
Maryland Institute for Emergency
Medical Services Systems
Baltimore, Maryland

Paul E. Pepe, M.D., F.A.C.E.P.
Director, City of Houston Emergency
Medical Services,
Associate Professor, Departments of
Medicine, Surgery and Pediatrics,
Baylor College of Medicine
Houston, Texas

Ronald G. Pirrallo, M.D.
SAEM Physio-Control Fellow in EMS,
Department of Emergency Medicine,
William Beaumont Hospital–Royal Oak
Royal Oak, Michigan

James Pointer, M.D.
Medical Director, City and County of
San Francisco Emergency Medical
Services Agency
San Francisco, California

Robert Pringle, Jr., NREMT–P
Firefighter/Paramedic,
Dale City Volunteer Fire & Rescue
Department
Woodbridge, Virginia

Ameen I. Ramzy, M.D.
Maryland State EMS Director,
Maryland Institute for Emergency
Medical Services Systems
Baltimore, Maryland

Steven J. Rottman, M.D., F.A.C.E.P.
Professor of Medicine,
Division of Emergency Medicine,
Director, UCLA Center for Prehospital
Care
Medical Director, City of Burbank EMS
Los Angeles, California

Robert A. Swor, D.O., F.A.C.E.P.
EMS Director,
William Beaumont Hospital–Royal Oak
Clinical Instructor,
Section of Emergency Medicine,
Department of Surgery,
University of Michigan
Royal Oak, Michigan

**Andrew G. Wilson, Jr., M.D.,
F.A.C.E.P.**
Chief, Department of Emergency
Medicine,
William Beaumont Hospital–Royal Oak
Royal Oak, Michigan

Barak Wolff, EMT–B, M.P.H.,
Chief, New Mexico Primary Care and
EMS Bureau
Santa Fe, New Mexico

Donald M. Yealy, M.D., F.A.C.E.P.
Senior Staff Physician and Director of
Research,
Department of Emergency Medicine,
Scott and White Memorial Hospital
Temple, Texas

Preface

In January 1991 the National Association of EMS Physicians sponsored a national meeting entitled "Quality Assurance in EMS" to address the burgeoning interest of evaluating emergency medical services (EMS). Neither the faculty nor the attendees ever envisioned the pace of change for this topic since that meeting. In prehospital care and in all of health care, there has been a dramatic revolution in the approach to improving quality.

The principles of Continuous Quality Improvement (CQI), which have been applied to industry in the United States, are now being applied to health care nationally. This "new approach" embodies good, old-fashioned principles of pride in workmanship, empowerment of front-line employees, commitment to excellence, demand for training, and emphasis on improving processes. Impressive strides have been made in health-care processes in selected hospitals across the country, although the effect of this new approach on direct patient care has yet to be documented.

How this new approach will impact EMS is another question entirely. Since the EMS act of 1973, prehospital care has evolved with an emphasis on a systems approach to patient care. This foundation should respond well to the CQI emphasis on processes. The emphasis of dependence on front-line providers is particularly important and well-suited to EMS. Prehospital patient care is rendered in the most uncontrolled circumstances in all of medicine, and emergency medical technicians (EMTs) and paramedics have to be empowered to control and improve their environment. In the matter of excellence, it is the considered opinion of these editors that there are no groups more dedicated to patient welfare than paramedics and EMTs. Whether any new management strategy can coordinate the strange bedfellows of dispatcher, police, fire, hospital, physicians, governmental resources, and others to *continually* improve EMS remains to be seen.

The contributing authors to this text discuss the state of the art of improving the quality of prehospital care. The first section of the text addresses the concepts of quality assurance, quality improvement, and implementation of change. Next, fundamental issues to program development (legal considerations, discipline, funding, data collection) are discussed. Approaches in a variety of EMS environments (urban, suburban, rural, air-medical, and trauma systems) are then presented. The final section addresses special roles in management and several different tools that have been used to improve care.

Readers will be disappointed if their purpose in using this text is to find a single program that can be applied to their EMS system. Quality management in health care is evolving rapidly, and many approaches and solutions will be offered in the years ahead. Our goal is to present the reader with the tools necessary to initiate and integrate the complex process of evaluating and effecting change in a specific EMS system. The success of any EMS system lies vested in the people who make up that system and their commitment to quality patient care. We hope that, through this text, those people will come away with the tools necessary to initiate the unending process of moving EMS systems toward excellence.

Chief Editor   Robert A. Swor, D.O.
Editors   Steven J. Rottman, M.D.
               Ronald G. Pirrallo, M.D.
               Eric Davis, M.D.

Acknowledgments

The creation of *Quality Management in Prehospital Care* is the result of the work of many individuals. Although much of the "credit" for this text will fall to the contributing authors and editors, we would like to recognize the efforts of many individuals without whom this book would not have been possible. Some of the individuals the editors would like to make special note of include:

Dr. Paul Paris for his initial wisdom to identify quality as a key issue to all of us in EMS

Ms. Katie Stage-Kern for her unfailing effort to develop a "Quality Assurance in EMS" program for the National Association of EMS Physicians

Dr. Ronald L. Krome for his enduring interest in supporting the pursuit of excellence in emergency care and his effort and unique ability to encourage this pursuit

Dr. Steve Davidson for his persistent challenging of what we do today, so that we may do better tomorrow

Ms. Nancy Peterson for her tireless work to keep this project on schedule and her neverending good humor in dealing with the complexities of this text

Ms. Claire Merrick and Mosby–Year Book, Inc., for their interest in developing *Quality Management in Prehospital Care*

Dr. Andrew Wilson for his encouragement, support, and the many hours spent discussing quality in EMS and how to pursue it

Ms. Sharonne Lucido for her faithful assistance and steady, sure performance in the face of a nervous editor

Messrs. Bob Elling, James Eastham, Jr., and Samuel Getz, Jr., for their careful and thoughtful reviews and editorial comments on this manuscript

Last, but clearly not least, the editors realize full well that a project such as this does not develop without the support, encouragement, tolerance, and understanding of our wives and families. We cannot thank them enough for their support.

Section One

Concepts in Quality Management

The ability to improve the quality of prehospital care requires an understanding of the approaches used to assess quality and implement changes. The authors in this section take varied approaches to their definitions of quality, quality assurance, and the application of industrial quality improvement to health care. Implementation of change in concept and in the hospital setting is presented because quality improvement in the prehospital setting is still in its infancy.

1

Quality Assurance in EMS

Gene W. Kallsen, M.D.

I worry whoever thought up the term ''quality control'' thought that if we didn't control it, it would get out of hand.

JANE WAGNER[33]

Quality assurance (QA) in health care has received a great deal of new attention in recent years. Although QA in emergency medical services (EMS) continues to be poorly standardized, it is finally becoming the subject of legitimate study.[30,32]

Although health-care providers have long been motivated to provide high-quality care, the current increased emphasis on QA is primarily driven by third-party payors and risk managers. Recent Health Care Financing Administration (HCFA) regulations state that it is the obligation of health-care practitioners to ensure that services rendered or ordered by them are provided economically, are of a quality meeting professionally recognized standards of care, and are supported by evidence of medical necessity and quality.[15] In the past, high quality in health care delivery was simply assumed; now it is required by federal regulation. Although the HCFA regulations do not specifically apply to prehospital care at this time, these regulations and others like them are spearheading a revolution in quality assessment and quality assurance throughout the health care industry.

The president of the Joint Commission on Accreditation of Healthcare Organizations (JCAHO), Dennis S. O'Leary, M.D., points out that[22]:

> The growing impatience of the government and others is evidenced by accelerated efforts to fill the quality assessment vacuum. Published hospital mortality rates and other alleged measures of quality, together with standardless evaluations of patient care, are prominent symptoms of the malaise. These efforts are patently crude and overly simplistic, but they serve affectively to cast the gauntlet before the physician community. We should understand clearly that cursing the darkness will not be a sufficient response.

What Is Quality?

Quality in health care is a concept that still lacks precise definition. Although noble attempts to define the term have been made by Rudstein[26] and Steffan,[29]

3

they disagree about whether quality of care should be measured by its outcome or its process.

In 1986, the House of Delegates to the American Medical Association (AMA) adopted a definition of quality of care that stated that other important elements, in addition to favorable outcome, can be used to identify care of high quality.[5] The AMA criteria include optimal improvement in the patient's physiologic status, physical function, emotional and intellectual performance, and comfort. The definition also emphasizes preventive medicine and early detection and treatment. High-quality care requires timely attention without delay and without unnecessary interruption. It seeks to achieve the informed cooperation and participation of the patient, and is based on accepted principles of medical science. Furthermore, such care is provided with sensitivity to the patient's stress and anxiety, and with concern for the patient's overall welfare. It makes efficient use of technology and other resources, and should be sufficiently documented in the patient's medical record to enable continuity of care. The very length of the AMA definition illustrates the complexity of the subject.

Avedis Donabedian has written classic treatises on the subject of QA. His definition of quality requires that some summation of benefits, risks, and costs must be considered.[11] He also notes that individual expectations and evaluations can affect the definition of the quality of care[12]:

> Before assessment begins we must decide how quality is to be defined, and that depends on whether one assesses only the performance of practitioners or also the contributions of patients in the health-care system; on how broadly health and responsibility for health are defined; on whether the maximally effective or optimally effective care is sought; and on whether individual or social preferences define the optimum.

Perhaps the most definitive statement on quality and medical care is provided by Dennis O'Leary[22]:

> We start with a struggle to define quality, as if our paralysis must continue until this task is completed. Although important, this is a potentially endless intellectual exercise, and medicine does not have the luxury of perpetual cerebral calisthenics. Ultimately, we will find that quality assessment, like the practice of medicine itself, is both science and art.

Quality Assurance Models in Health Care

Donabedian's QA model involves assessment of structure, process, and outcome. *Structure* refers to the attributes of the settings in which care is provided. *Process* refers to what is actually done when giving or receiving care, including the patient's and the practitioner's activities. *Outcome* refers to the effects of care on the health status of the patient and the population. The patient's degree of satisfaction and changes in the patient's knowledge and behavior are included under a broad definition of health-status outcome.[12]

Donabedian also points out that using structure and process parameters as part of the QA process is valid only to the extent that good structure results in good process, which in turn results in good outcome. "It is necessary therefore to have established such a relationship before any particular component of structure process or outcome can be used to assess quality."[12]

The JCAHO has been the primary federally sanctioned health-care QA organization for decades. Although accreditation by the JCAHO is voluntary for its 5000 member hospitals, such accreditation serves as the typical route for qualification for receipt of Medicare funds. The organization has been under pressure from its member hospitals who complain that structure and process criteria are not well linked to outcome. At the same time, other critics have asserted that the JCAHO has failed to demand uniform high-quality care.

In 1986, the JCAHO began the "Agenda for Change" under the leadership of Dennis O'Leary.[18] Measurement of "Does this organization provide quality health care?" instead of "Can this organization provide quality health care?" became the goal. Expert panels were created to identify and select clinical indicators that could be directly related to outcome. If structure or process indicators were included, they would have to show a demonstrated relationship to outcome. QA research and developmental activities included in the Agenda for Change were the identification and selection of clinical indicators, identification and selection of organizational and management indicators, development of risk-adjustment methods, establishment of an ongoing monitoring and evaluation process, and modification of survey and accreditation procedures.

A clinical indicator, as described by the JCAHO, is a defined, measurable dimension of the appropriateness of an important aspect of patient care; examples include deaths, hospital-acquired infections, and adverse reactions. It is emphasized that clinical indicators are not direct indicators of quality but are instead to be used as screens to identify cases that need in-depth professional scrutiny. Additionally, clinical indicators are of two types. *Sentinel* indicators require that every case be individually examined. For example, an unrecognized esophageal placement of an endotracheal tube is a sentinel event. *Rate* indicators, on the other hand, require further examination only if the frequency occurs outside of the expected range. Inability to successfully place an endotracheal tube in the prehospital setting is acceptable a small percentage of the time, although unrecognized malposition as evidenced in the first example is not.

More recently, the JCAHO has emphasized the concept of continuous quality improvement (CQI) instead of QA.[21] This intentional transition appears to be based only in part on the semantics of the term quality assurance—quality can never be assured, but it can be improved. There are, however, fundamental differences between CQI and QA that will be discussed more fully in the text that follows.

CQI demands an integrated approach to quality, involvement of the entire organization, empowerment of front-line personnel to be active in the process of change, and commitment by management to expend energy and resources to effect necessary changes. It also emphasizes the *processes* involved in the provision of care rather than specifically reviewing care rendered by individuals. Although the JCAHO does not yet require CQI to be implemented in hospitals, it requires that by 1992 hospital administrations be educated in the principles of CQI.[17] This shift in "quality management" philosophy and methodology will doubtless have a fundamental impact on how health care is rendered in the prehospital setting.

The American College of Emergency Physicians has published an excellent QA manual for emergency medicine edited by Schneiderman and Wiseman.[27] Although this manual is primarily directed at the hospital emergency department, its step-by-step approach to QA can be adapted to prehospital care.

Quality Assurance in EMS

A reasonable QA model in EMS can evolve from the previously discussed models. The QA provider must first achieve a level of authority that allows participation across agency and provider boundaries.[16] Goals must be established and mutually agreed to. Methods must be implemented to evaluate compliance with those goals. And, finally, a feedback system must be created to provide a correction and redirection toward the established goals. Cooper has described the importance of the EMS system's approach to QA.[10]

The establishment of goals is a generic concept that transcends the jargon of QA. Whether goals are called "clinical indicators," "screens," or some other QA terms, they must be established through a reasonable process and must be implemented only after a reasonable consensus has been reached. Goals can be driven by specific laws or regulations, by the standards or guidelines of professional organizations, by recent research, or by the use of the experience of other systems. Draft goals should be articulated, negotiated, synthesized, and finally adopted.

Schneiderman[27] cites the importance of participation and acceptance by the medical staff for all screens that are used in the emergency department. The JCAHO relies heavily on expert panels to establish its clinical indicators. Donabedian and Steffan both suggest that the values and goals of the patients themselves have an effect on what is a legitimate medical goal. Steffan[29] provides a fascinating discussion of the process of goal setting. Doctors tend to rely heavily on the goal of getting the patient well, whereas patients put more emphasis on goals such as preserving dignity, maintaining choices, and keeping costs down.

Goals or standards relating to patient outcome are of potentially more value than structure or process goals. Eisenberg[13] illustrates how outcome of cardiac arrest can measure a system's quality; Boyd[6] reports how outcomes can measure trauma systems; and Shackford[28] describes how a medical audit committee has successfully applied outcome QA to a trauma system. A number of publications specify goals or standards, usually of the structure or process type, that can be applied to prehospital care.[1-3,7,9,23-25,31]

Whichever process is used to establish legitimate goals, development of consensus regarding those goals and "selling" the goals systemwide are essential to success. Broad participation in goalsetting makes the task of goalselling much easier.

Once the goals are established, compliance should be measured. Tools of measurement include simple observation, continual measurement, intermittent measurement (such as random chart audits), and exception reporting (such as incident reports). The range of data system options is beyond the scope of this discussion. Suffice it to say that the data-collection instrument needs to be designed to allow sufficient measurement of achievement of the goal. A common error is to attempt to collect thorough, detailed data on all aspects of the system and all aspects of patient care; this frequently results in a system of "garbage in, garbage out" yielding little or no meaningful data. Careful intermittent sampling is often the preferable choice.

Finally, a feedback system is needed to create change when there is a disparity between goals and performance. Change is best achieved through positive feedback and is usually only slowly, painfully (if ever) achieved through negative feedback alone. Individuals who perform in keeping with established goals deserve frequent and sometimes public recognition and awards. Public information and education need to emphasize the goals and achievements of the emergency services system in terms that the public can easily understand and support. Key policymakers, such as politicians, need very specific information about positive aspects of the system and their own role in system development.

When goals are not being met, system change and policy clarification are more often appropriate steps than disciplinary action against personnel. Morale is best in systems in which prehospital personnel sense that the system is willing to learn, adjust, and evolve as problems arise rather than find yet another individual scapegoat for each "incident."

The Role of Leadership

EMS systems are still in their infancy and continue to evolve rapidly. QA, as a specific component of EMS systems, is undeveloped, poorly standardized, and still unfolding. Change and the need for change are everywhere. As a result, both the urgency and the opportunity for leadership abound.

Kotter recently differentiated between leadership and management as follows[19]: Management is about coping with complexity, whereas leadership is about coping with change. Management deals with complexity by planning, budgeting, organizing, staffing, controlling, and problem solving. Leadership deals with change by setting a direction, and aligning, motivating, and inspiring people. Managers work through the chain of command and pay close attention to organizational charts. Leaders align forces throughout the organization and inspire and motivate them, rallying them around new goals and system changes. Leaders articulate the organization's vision in a manner that stresses an audience's values. Leaders involve people in deciding how to achieve the organization's vision, provide coaching feedback, and become role models. Leaders help people to grow professionally and to enhance both their own career and their self-esteem. Finally, leaders recognize and reward success.

David Halberstam describes the evolution of the American and Japanese auto industries over the last four decades in his book, *The Reckoning*.[14] The American auto industry was not only one of the most incredible success stories in history, its mass production of high-quality vehicles revolutionized our culture and our world. Eventually, though, its prominence and its quality were in many ways surpassed by the Japanese automobile industry.

Halberstam chronicles some of the events leading up to this dramatic reversal. The selection of goals and the quality control (QC) process contributed to that reversal. The early leadership in the American automobile industry consisted of bright engineers who were obsessed with the dream of creating a quality automobile. Henry Ford, for one, personally designed and created automobiles and introduced mass production to the automobile industry. Eventually, the top leadership positions in the American automobile industry were filled with people who had training in finance and economics and knew little or nothing about the product itself. Worse still, they often lacked the passion for automobiles that characterized people such as Ford.

With the change in this leadership came a dramatic change in organizational goalsetting. The industry became more obsessed with making money than with making automobiles. The stock became the product, and the value of the stock became more important than the quality of the automobile. Finally, the QC process itself changed. Whereas quality had once been an essential part of the vision, QC became a mere component—one that could be delegated.

When the automobile industry rediscovered quality in recent years, W. Edwards Deming became one of its gurus. Ironically, Deming was virtually unknown in American industry during the 1950s when he was a national hero in Japan. His technical message of carefully measured and carefully controlled tolerances complements his organizational message that quality must be central to the organization's mission and must reign throughout the organization.

Deming stresses that this commitment to quality must start at the top. A telling anecdote that illustrates this issue involved a Ford Motor Company vice president who requested that Deming work with the company to improve QA. Deming declined, indicating that he would be willing to talk with Ford only when the company *president* committed to quality management and personally requested his services. This commitment to quality "from the top" must be translated into a change in the "organizational culture," as defined by Deming and others, in which all employees learn and adhere to the organizational commitment to quality.

Leadership in EMS

Quality EMS systems have developed in this country through the inspired leadership of physician medical directors. Physician leaders have articulated a vision of medical excellence and nurtured developing systems to provide quality care. To suggest, however, that these systems developed solely because of physician input would be shortsighted. EMS systems are similar in structure to hospital systems and need both medical and administrative leadership to be effective.

Because the role of EMS systems is providing medical care, physicians must be intimately involved in the delivery of that care. Krentz[20] argues that the role of the physician medical director is to be the system's patient advocate. Development of standards of practice, medical protocols, education, and evaluation are all critical roles of the physician. The physician must be intimately acquainted with the capabilities and limitations within the prehospital setting and the providers of care at all levels. He must be a student of the medical literature and facilitate changes in the EMS system that correspond to the evolution of medical practice. He must also be able to articulate the medical value of the system to both the medical community and the population at large.

Toward that end, the medical director must be an integral component (and supporter) of the system used to evaluate and improve care. He must also be able to ensure the quality of that quality improvement process to facilitate the EMS system's maturation. The extent of the physicians' activities must not be limited to medical issues only, since the system structure must also be capable of providing quality care. Adequate protocols, personnel, and training are of no medical benefit unless a vehicle is available to arrive in a timely fashion at the bedside of a patient in ventricular fibrillation.

Similarly, the EMS system administrator, fire chief, company owner, and other administrative heads must take a leadership role in quality EMS care. Resources must be procured and priorities established to create a system of excellence. Personnel, equipment, management expertise, and interrelationships with supporting organizations must all be in place for the system to thrive. The administration must also review medical issues to determine that they are practical as well as medically sound. There must be administrative support to supply the substantial resources needed to develop and carry out a quality improvement program, and the administration must be willing to commit resources to improve the problems identified. In short, a partnership must be developed between the medical and administrative structures for the system to evolve into one of high quality.

Legal Issues in Quality Assurance

Several legal issues are relevant to the QA process. Laws concerning QA fit into three broad categories: authorization, immunity for witnesses and peer groups, and immunity from discovery. See Chapter 8 for a further discussion of these topics.

Authorization

The authority to initiate QA activities must first be clearly delegated to the appropriate individuals within the system. Typically, the legislation that covers the development of EMS systems state by state has assigned QA responsibility and authority to an individual, usually to a medical director. It is essential that the authority exists, that it is commensurate with the responsibility, and that its delegation is clear.[16]

Immunity for Witnesses and Peer Groups

Several states have passed legislation that grants immunity from civil damage for peer-review activities and testimony. For example, the applicable section of the California code states that there is "no monetary liability for professional society or member of society for any act or proceeding undertaken or performed . . . to maintain the professional standards of the society. . . ."[8] This section applies to physicians, dentists, dental hygienists, podiatrists, registered dieticians, chiropractors, optometrists, veterinarians, and psychologists, but not to paramedics. Clearly, such provisions should be extended to prehospital peer-review processes in which they currently do not apply.

Immunity from Discovery

We may wish that our systems would never be involved in any kind of litigation and that all quality issues could be handled internally. Society, however, relies heavily on the tort system to correct perceived injustices. As flawed as that system may be, we must remember that the plaintiff's attorney will continue to have access to the facts surrounding a case of alleged negligence.

Although it is not an achievable goal to prevent a plaintiff's attorney from discovering the facts of the case, it is reasonable to prevent them from accessing the details and conclusions of the peer-review process and the QA process. Even though legislators have granted this type of immunity to hospital QA committees, the extent to which this immunity includes prehospital QA varies from state to state.

Confidentiality in the peer-review process is important for a number of reasons. It protects individuals from unnecessary embarrassment. Lawsuits that would otherwise have never been initiated often result from gossip within the EMS community concerning both the details of the case (violating patient confidentiality) and the details of the peer-review or medical director findings. These violations of confidentiality can themselves void the immunity from discovery in certain circumstances.

The goal of immunity from discovery must be put into perspective. It has been suggested that QA programs should be suspended or not initiated until further immunity from discovery can be ensured. Experience to date, however, does not justify such a position. More important, QA is far too critical to defer. Still, it must be done carefully and with full understanding of the limitations to immunity in your state.

Personnel Issues

In 1988, the AMA's Council on Medical Service adopted "Guidelines for Quality Assurance."[4] This 10-point position outlines several excellent principles, which emphasize education and remediation rather than discipline. It also addresses principles to be taken into consideration any time action is considered or taken against professional medical personnel.

The AMA's principles include the need to involve those professionals in the development of the policies and processes, to apply the process objectively and impartially, to trigger remedial activity based on concern for overall practice patterns rather than single cases, and to institute remedial actions only *after* direct discussions with the practitioner involved. These guidelines further stress that when practitioners are not responsive to remedial activities, restrictions or disciplinary actions should be imposed. Imposing such restriction or discipline needs to be timely and consistent with due process. The QA process should be structured and operated so as to ensure immunity for the practitioners conducting or applying such systems. Finally, QA systems should recognize care of high quality and correct instances of deficient practice.

A few words about "paper trails" are appropriate at this point. The due process of any personnel action requires careful and complete written documentation. However, if the discoverability of QA findings is in any question in your state, carefully consider how much written documentation is necessary and sufficient for QA activities.

Scope of Quality Assurance Activities

All of us have limited time and resources for QA activities. Therefore, we must carefully consider and prioritize the appropriate scope of such activities. I urge you to consider expanding your QA process into neglected areas at the same time that you consider limiting your scope to reduce duplication.

Although QA for paramedics is generally at least attempted, QA for emergency medical technicians (EMTs) is often less clear or even totally absent. Dispatchers, first responders, and "nonemergency" ambulance services are all areas for QA consideration. Unfortunately, you may find yourself limited in terms of authority. Again, the enabling legislation must clearly delegate the authority for QA for these levels to accountable medical personnel.

The QA process must not become bogged down with cases over which it has no jurisdiction. Some paramedics would like nothing better than for the EMS medical director to solve all the problems in nursing homes. It is better to direct nursing home complaints to the appropriate licensing agency, while reserving our time and resources for problems that fall under our authority. Likewise, paramedic-generated complaints about physicians are often turned over to the chief of their emergency department or, in extreme cases, to the state physician licensing agency. These should all be screened by the medical director, and individual judgment is important. Finally, the interagency QA process should steer personality conflicts back to individual agencies for their resolution.

Summary

The provision of quality care in EMS is the central critical issue concerning system leaders and all individual professionals working within that system. A good EMS system includes individuals who have shared in the process of developing QA goals or standards and who share a vision of what constitutes high quality care.

Processes that measure compliance with those standards must be fair and impartial, and remediation and reeducation are always preferable to disciplinary action. When discipline is necessary, it should carefully comply with all the principles and laws of due process. The scope of QA activities should be sufficiently wide to include essentially all components of EMS and sufficiently restricted so as to reduce duplication and cooperate with other regulatory agencies. We must continue to lobby for appropriate laws and regulations that allow clear authorization for the imposition of QA, provide immunity for individuals who participate in peer-review activities, and grant immunity from discovery for QA activities. Even without ideal legal protections, we must provide appropriate QA with documentation that is necessary and sufficient for the circumstances.

REFERENCES

1. American College of Emergency Physicians: Guidelines for emergency medical services systems, *Ann Emerg Med* 16:459-463, 1987.
2. American College of Emergency Physicians: Guidelines for trauma care systems, *Ann Emerg Med* 16:459-463, 1987.
3. American College of Surgeons: Committee on trauma (resource for optimal care of the injured patient—an update), *Am Coll Surg Bull* 75:20-29, 1989.
4. American Medical Association Council on Medical Service: Guidelines for quality assurance, *JAMA*, 259:2572, 1988.
5. American Medical Association Council on Medical Service: Quality of care, *JAMA* 256:1032-1034, 1986.
6. Boyd CR, Tolson MA, Copes WS: Evaluating trauma care: the TRISS method, *J Trauma* 27:370-378, 1987.
7. Cales RH: *Medical evaluation.* In Cales RH, Heilig RW, editors: *Trauma care systems,* Rockville, MD, 1986, Aspen Publishers.
8. Cal. Civ. Code para. 43.7.
9. Clawson JJ, Dernocoeur KB: *Principles of emergency medical dispatch,* Englewood Cliffs, N.J., 1988, Prentice Hall.
10. Cooper GF, Murrin P, Sheridan-McArdle M: Advances in quality assurance, *Advances in Trauma and Critical Care,* ed 2, St. Louis, 1987, Mosby—Year Book.

11. Donabedian A: *The definition of quality and approaches to its assessment,* Ann Arbor, Mich, 1980, Health Administration Press.
12. Donabedian A: *The quality of care: how can it be assessed? JAMA* 260:1743-1748, 1988.
13. Eisenberg M et al: Evaluation of paramedic programs using outcomes of prehospital resuscitation for cardiac arrest, *J Am Coll Emerg Physicians* 8:458-461, 1979.
14. Halberstam D: *The reckoning,* New York, 1986, Avon Books.
15. Health Care Financing Administration Regulations, *Federal Register,* vol 50, no 74, 474.30, April 17, 1985.
16. Holroyd BR, Knopp R, Kallsen G: Medical control: quality assurance in prehospital care, *JAMA* 256:1027-1031, 1986.
17. Joint Commission on Accreditation of Healthcare Organizations: *Accreditation manual for hospitals, 1992,* Chicago, 1992, The Commission.
18. Joint Commission on the Accreditation of Healthcare Organizations: Overview of the joint commission's agenda for change, August 1987 (unpublished).
19. Kotter JP: What leaders really do, *Harvard Business Review* 168(3):103-111, 1990.
20. Krentz MJ, Wainscott MP: Medical accountability, *Emerg Med Clin North Am,* February 17-33, 1990.
21. O'Leary DS: CQI—a step beyond QA: Joint Commission perspectives, Joint Commission on the Accreditation of Healthcare Organizations, March 1990.
22. O'Leary DS: Quality assessment: moving from theory to practice, *JAMA* 260:1760, September 1988.
23. Pepe PE, Stewart RD: Role of the physician in the prehospital setting, *Ann Emerg Med* 15:1480-1483, 1986.
24. Pointer JE: The advanced life support base hospital audit for medical control in an emergency medical services system, *Ann Emerg Med* 16:557-560, 1987.
25. Pons PT et al: The field instructor program: quality control of prehospital care, the first step, *J Emerg Med* 2:421-427, 1985.
26. Rutstein DD et al: Measuring the quality of medical care, *N Engl J Med* 294:582-588, 1976.
27. Schneiderman N, Wiseman M, editors: Quality assurance manual for emergency medicine, Dallas, 1987, American College of Emergency Physicians.
28. Shackford SR et al: Assuring quality in a trauma system—the medical audit committee: composition, cost, and results, *J Trauma* 27:866-875, 1987.
29. Steffan GE: Quality medical care: a definition, *JAMA* 260:56-61, 1988.
30. Stewart RB et al: A computer assisted quality assurance system for an emergency medical service, *Ann Emerg Med* 14:25-29, 1985.
31. Stout JL: Stout's standards of excellence for prehospital EMS systems, *J Emerg Med Serv* 1983.
32. Swor RA, Hoelzer M: A computer assisted quality assurance audit in a multiprovider EMS system, *Ann Emerg Med* 19:286-290, 1990.
33. Wagner J: *The search for signs of intelligent life in the universe,* New York, 1986, Harper & Row.

2

Concepts in EMS Quality Management

Richard M. McDowell, M.D.

Management of an emergency medical services (EMS) system involves the coordination of many system components. An effective quality assurance (QA) program requires coordination among the QA programs for each system component. Traditional QA methods in virtually every industry, including EMS, are being challenged and replaced with the newer concept of continuous quality improvement (CQI).

QA programs in the health-care industry have historically been viewed negatively by providers. They perceive that QA programs are imposed upon them and that the purpose of QA is to find mistakes made by providers. The principles of CQI have a fundamentally different emphasis than traditional QA programs and should apply exceptionally well to EMS systems. CQI teaches that improvements in patient care result from improvements in the entire system, rather than from better performance by providers; this "systems approach" fits well with the EMS system approach to patient care. These improvements, however, require a coordinated commitment from system managers and providers.

The goal of systemwide quality improvement (QI) of EMS is to improve patient care. This is best accomplished by understanding current quality management principles in general, current EMS quality issues in particular, and how to design a program's structure and content to ensure effective implementation.

This chapter discusses different aspects of systemwide QI: how it differs from traditional QA; how it differs from QA programs for individual components; how it is necessary to integrate the QA programs of the components; and, finally, how to accomplish this integration effectively.

EMS Systems versus Components

In 1973 the EMS Systems Act outlined 15 components of an EMS system. This federal legislation was intended to guide the development of state and regional EMS systems and to help fund them. Since then, there has been at least one revision to this original list of components to modernize it to emphasize different areas, such as medical control.[18] These two lists of EMS components are compared in Table 2-1.

Regardless of which set of components is ultimately chosen, the system must be managed as a whole, and the components must work together for the entire system to be effective. No one component or group of components should drive the system. For example, EMS components such as hospitals, which are both receiving facilities and specialty care units, represent powerful political entities. Transport agencies or communications facilities may also be politically powerful. Some of these components may resist outside influence and review. Others may try to function independently or to drive the system for purposes other than

Table 2-1. Components of an EMS System

Original	Revision
1. Manpower	—
2. Training	1. Training
3. Communications	2. Communications
4. Transportation	3. Prehospital transport agencies
	4. Interfacility transport agencies
5. Emergency facilities	5. Receiving facilities
6. Critical care units	6. Specialty care units
7. Public safety agencies	—
8. Consumer participation	—
9. Access to care	—
10. Patient transfer	—
11. Standardized recordkeeping	—
12. Public information and education	7. Public information and education
13. System review and evaluation	8. Audit and QA
14. Disaster	9. Disaster
15. Mutual aid	10. Mutual aid
	11. Protocols (triage, treatment, transport, transfer)
	12. Financing
	13. Dispatch
	14. Medical direction

quality patient care. Cooperation and coordination among all the components must be developed for a QA program to be effective. Responsibility for system management must rest with a lead agency that has the authority and responsibility for CQI of the entire system.

Any system composed of multiple components has the ability to integrate the individual component's quality management programs. Specific examples include a state EMS system, a city or county EMS system, or even a large single EMS service that interacts with many different receiving hospitals, command hospitals, first responders, and basic life support (BLS) and advanced life support (ALS) units.

General Quality Assurance Principles

Several models or principles of QA have been well described and applied in health care. These should be understood because of their historical importance and widespread applications. The three models discussed in this section are: (1) Donabedian's concept of structure/process/outcome; (2) the American Medical Association (AMA) guidelines for professional peer review; and (3) the Joint Commission on Accreditation of Healthcare Organizations' (JCAHO) monitoring and evaluation process.

Donabedian

Avedis Donabedian[6] is the father of classical medical QA. His model for classifying information about the quality of patient care has pervaded the QA literature in health care.[7] Donabedian's model uses three categories: structure, process, and outcome.

Structure refers to the settings in which care occurs, including the organizational structure as well as the resources, both material and human. In EMS, structural elements that could be the focus of QA include ambulances, equipment, manpower, training, communications, and receiving facilities. For example, ambulances should meet certain specifications and requirements and undergo inspection and a certification process. Emergency medical technicians (EMTs) should meet certain selection requirements, including having graduated from an approved training curriculum taught by an approved faculty. Communication centers should meet certain hardware requirements and demonstrate performance capabilities, which might include time standards for handling calls and use of prearrival instructions. Receiving facilities should undergo inspection and certification to demonstrate that adequate personnel, equipment, and systems are available to receive EMS patients.

Process refers to the care that the patient receives, including how the patient seeks care and how the practitioner delivers that care. In EMS, process elements that could be the focus of QA include dispatching; medical care in the field; nonmedical decisions made by EMTs in the field, such as not to transport or to sign against medical advice, and triage decisions, such as trauma center transports. Each of these process elements is represented as a protocol, which should be used as guidelines to monitor treatment. For example, field care should be examined using treatment protocols; nonmedical protocols, such as refusal-of-care protocols; and adherence to trauma-triage protocols. In addition, dispatching protocols and adherence to prearrival instructions can be examined.

Outcome refers to the effects of care on the health status of patients and populations. In EMS, outcome elements that could be the focus of QA include trauma registries and cardiac-arrest outcome data. These two examples represent the final outcome of patients who may pass through several areas of care that are not directly controlled by the EMS system. Some experts suggest that outcomes for an EMS system should focus on results of field therapy only, with all measurement occurring in the emergency department before any additional hospital intervention. However, it is difficult to identify meaningful outcome elements that can help improve EMS care when outcomes are measured in emergency departments only. Identifying important and pertinent outcome studies for EMS systems has been extremely difficult.

Donabedian's model is based on the premise that good structure should increase the likelihood of good process, which should in turn increase the likelihood of good outcome. Although this sounds reasonable, does this hold true for EMS or for any other system in which it has been applied? EMS has traditionally emphasized structure and process and almost completely excluded outcome studies, in part because they have been difficult to identify.

AMA Guidelines

The AMA has published guidelines for peer review in QA (see box on page 18). How does peer review in EMS relate to the concept of medical control? Are they mutually exclusive? Holroyd and others[13] have written that "medical control is a system of physician-directed quality assurance. . . ." This does not mean, however, that critical concepts of peer review should be excluded. A comprehensive and reasonable plan for quality management of an EMS system must include peer review by providers. Although most of these guidelines may be adapted for use in EMS QA programs, a few are of particular note:

1. EMTs should be involved with the development and implementation of QA programs.
2. In general, remedial activity should focus on patterns of practice rather than on individual deviations from protocol. A "QA note" to a generally excellent medic regarding a single failed or delayed intubation usually serves no useful purpose in upgrading patient care. It may, however, sour that medic's view of the purpose and usefulness of the QA program.
3. Emphasis should be on education and retraining rather than on sanctions, which should be reserved for situations in which it is necessary to protect the public. QA notes to good providers with occasional deviations from protocol should be supplanted by discovery of trends in patient care that identify a provider who needs retraining. Medical control should use sanctions when necessary to protect the public.

American Medical Association Guidelines for Quality Assurance

- The general policies and processes to be used in any QA activity should be developed and concurred with by the professionals whose performance will be scrutinized and should be objectively and impartially administered.
- Any remedial QA activity related to an individual practitioner should be triggered by concern for that individual's overall practice patterns rather than by deviation from specified criteria in single cases.
- The institution of any remedial activity should be preceded by discussion with the practitioner involved.
- Emphasis should be placed on education and modification of unacceptable practice patterns rather than on sanctions.
- The QA system should make available the appropriate educational resources needed to effect desired practice modifications.
- Feedback mechanisms should be established to monitor and document needed changes in practice patterns.
- Restrictions or disciplinary actions should be imposed on those practitioners not responsive to remedial activities, whenever the appropriate professional peers deem such action necessary to protect the public.
- The imposition of restrictions or discipline should be timely and consistent with due process.
- QA systems should be structured and operated so as to ensure immunity for practitioners conducting or applying such systems who are acting in good faith.
- QA systems should be structured to recognize care of high quality as well as to correct instances of deficient practice.

JCAHO Recommendations

The JCAHO[12] published a 10-step monitoring and evaluation process designed to help health-care organizations manage the quality of the care they provide. This process has become a standard model that is used almost universally in hospital QA systems and has firmly introduced several terms and concepts into the QA lexicon. The terms *indicators* and *thresholds* are joined with *scope of care*, which has come to be called *standards*. Now the phrase *standards/indicators/ thresholds* is used routinely in QA. These 10 steps (see box) form a feedback loop when diagrammed together, which is a critical QA concept.

The definitions of standards/indicators/thresholds referred to here should be considered together, as three parts of one important QA concept. A standard is a generalized goal that is an achievable model of excellence and is used to define expectations. An indicator is an objective behavior or outcome that can be measured to determine compliance with a standard. A threshold is an established level or percentage of acceptable compliance that indicates when further evaluation should be initiated; this is usually less than 100%, thus

---

Joint Commission on Accreditation of Healthcare Organizations' 10-Step Quality Assurance Process

1. Assign responsibility
2. Delineate scope of care
3. Identify important aspects of care
4. Identify indicators
5. Establish thresholds for evaluation
6. Collect and organize data
7. Evaluate care
8. Take actions to solve problems
9. Assess actions and document improvement
10. Communicate relevant information to the organizationwide QA program

---

removing the burden of the term standard as a result of clinical exceptions in established guidelines.

In summary, these three traditional models of QA all contain important principles that can be applied to EMS quality management. Each defines a method by which EMS systems may be analyzed.

Continuous Quality Improvement

CQI is replacing traditional methods of QA in many American companies. Although sometimes referred to as total quality management or by other terms, CQI is very different from traditional QA.

A brief history of CQI is helpful to put it into perspective for health care and EMS. The concept began in a limited number of industries in the United States around the 1930s and was pioneered by men such as W. Edwards Deming and Joseph Juran. In the 1950s, Japanese leaders invited Deming to introduce this concept to post–World War II Japanese companies. His teachings were embraced throughout that country's ravaged economy and have been credited with the dramatic turnaround in the meaning of the phrase "made in Japan." His name is still prominent in Japan, where a national Deming award is associated with excellence and quality.

In the 1980s renewed interest in the success of Deming's philosophy in Japan brought him back into American industry to teach his management principles.[5,20] Now there are growing numbers of manufacturing and service industries in the United States that have been using CQI for nearly a decade. These ideas are also being taught by others such as Philip Crosby,[4] who began his Quality College for business executives in 1979. New concepts of quality management are taught.

The history of CQI in health care dates from the late 1980s/early 1990s, with the prominent leader Donald Berwick[3] of the Harvard Community Health Plan. Hospitals throughout the country are applying this new quality process with encouraging improvements in operational aspects of patient care. Whether this method can be applied to the complex decision-making of patient care remains to be determined.[21] In EMS, experience is even more limited. In the first half of 1991, however, three national EMS quality conferences included CQI as a significant topic. These conferences were sponsored by the National Association of EMS Physicians (NAEMSP), the American College of Emergency Physicians (ACEP), and Jems Communications, Inc.

This section presents a brief outline of Deming's management method as an introduction to the concept of CQI. A more comprehensive discussion will follow in Chapter 6.

Deming teaches his management method as 14 points, adding several "deadly diseases" and some obstacles that typically prevent Western management from implementing these points. These 14 points are as follows:

1. Create constancy of purpose for the improvement of product and service. Long-term investments must be made in research, education, innovation, and continuous improvement.
2. Adopt the new philosophy. Management must be transformed and perhaps some structures dismantled so that quality becomes the new "religion."
3. Cease dependence on mass inspection. Inspection to find mistakes is too late. Inspection is to monitor a process, not to create quality; quality comes from improving the process.
4. End the practice of awarding business based on the price tag alone. Price has no meaning without a measure of the quality being purchased.
5. Improve constantly and forever the system of production and service. Finding a point of variance and its cause and then removing it only puts the process back to where it was in the first place; it does not improve the process.
6. Institute training and retraining. It is difficult to erase improper training.
7. Institute leadership. In hiring personnel, management takes responsibility for their success or failure. Most people who do poorly are not malingerers but have been misplaced.
8. Drive out fear. People are often afraid to point out problems or admit a mistake.
9. Break down barriers between staff areas. There must be teamwork and everyone must share the same goals for the entire company; the tone for this is set by management.
10. Eliminate slogans, exhortations, and targets for the workforce. The phrases "zero defects" and "do it right the first time" imply that the problem is the worker, not the system.
11. Eliminate numeric quotas. Remember that haste makes waste; piece work can guarantee inefficiency and high cost for rework by including

allowances for defective items. This applies to management also, since all goals should be set with an accompanying plan to accomplish them.

12. Remove barriers to pride in workmanship. Examples include poor instructions about the job, poor tools and materials, changing standards, arbitrary or poorly trained supervisors, and no feedback until a subjective yearly performance rating.

13. Institute a vigorous program of education and retraining. This investment in people is required for the achievement of long-term goals.

14. Take action to accomplish the transformation. Management must have the courage to change to continuous improvement, and there must be a critical mass of people to effect that change.

EMS should be committed to the principles of CQI at the highest administrative levels. In addition, these principles must be taught to providers at all levels, all of whom must understand and embrace these principles to effect change and continuous improvement.

Comparison of Quality Assurance with Continuous Quality Improvement

The previous section on general QA principles presented a broad picture of traditional methods using three widely used models. The section on the Deming management method showed how a broad subject like CQI can be approached using 14 specific principles of management. Although it is not easy to compare these widely divergent methods directly, this section offers some comparisons. Real understanding of the differences between QA and CQI, however, requires the study of both systems.

System Problems versus People Problems

One of the biggest differences between CQI and QA is that CQI focuses on system problems whereas QA focuses on people problems. Leaders in CQI write that 80% to 85% of quality problems are due to the system, whereas only 15% to 20% are because of people. CQI teaches that it is important to look at how people are hired, trained, and supervised, and then at how the entire system functions to allow people to do their jobs well. The system must remove obstacles that inhibit job performance and supply people with what they need to do their jobs well.

Management Responsibility versus Provider Responsibility

The CQI focus on improving the system rather than blaming people for problems places more responsibility on management than traditional QA. In CQI it is incumbent on management to hire, train, and supervise the right people, and then put them into a process that can allow them to get their jobs done. Problems are to be solved by management, not blamed on people.

Prospective and Constructive versus Retrospective and Punitive

QA relies heavily on inspection of a process, whereas in CQI, this is just one of several tools to study a process. QA uses inspection to enforce minimum standards and identify problems that need to be solved. This means that QA is perceived as punitive. This retrospective inspection identifies defects that are caused by some error in the process, to which blame is attached. This faultfinding is often directed toward people. Problems identified trigger negative feedback. On the other hand, CQI is designed to look at a process from the very beginning to find opportunities for improvement. CQI also inspects processes, but when defects are found they are analyzed using statistical principles. If the defects are statistically significant, they are considered to be opportunities for improving the process.

Retrospective review and inspection of a process is a technique that needs to be used even in the most advanced CQI program. When used appropriately, this is an important statistical way to monitor a process to identify areas in which improvement is needed. Unfortunately, this has become the overwhelming focus of traditional QA and has lost its statistical context. This aspect of traditional QA should not be discarded but rather used as a tool in a strategy of overall quality management.

Standards

In QA, standards are generalized goals that are achievable models of excellence used to define expectations. Although usually intended to be minimum QA standards, they tend to become ceilings. These standards are used to inspect a process for defects. Indicators and thresholds are used to monitor minimum standards and correct unwarranted deviations. In effect, QA polices a system to enforce minimum standards. In CQI, standards are based on best-practice models that are emulated throughout the system.

Consider a bell-shaped curved that represents performance of an EMS system (see Figure 2-1). The curve has a median value, and improvement in system performance is represented as a higher value for the median. In QA the system is inspected for poor performance, which is represented by the tail of the bell-shaped curve. When this tail is removed, the median of the curve is shifted only slightly since the area under the tail is so small. This represents only a small improvement in system performance. In CQI the system is improved not by inspection but by continuous alterations to cause emulation of best-practice models. This causes the median to shift upward and the bell-shaped curve to become more narrow around the median. Not only is median performance improved, but variation in performance is also decreased. This results in a

QUALITY IMPROVEMENT

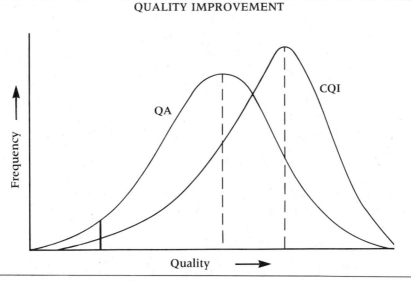

Figure 2-1 CQI works to improve performance of all providers, not just outliers at the low end of the curve.

much more significant improvement in the system that uses CQI than the one that uses QA.

Traditional Quality Assurance as a Subset of Continuous Quality Improvement

Traditional QA activities have played an important role in improving EMS systems and should not be discarded. Rather, these programs of retrospective audit and review should be recognized as a subset of the much broader CQI program. CQI teaches that processes should be measured and studied; this is the role that traditional QA has performed in EMS. It must be understood, however, that addressing individual outliers will not necessarily cause significant improvement in the system of care.[22] QA has served as an effective problem-*identifying* mechanism in EMS. Analysis of problems and methods of problem *solving* are the emphasis of CQI.

EMS System–based versus EMS Component–based Quality Assurance

The concept of categorizing EMS QA into both system-based and component-based elements is derived from QA guidelines for trauma patients. It is important to understand both elements so they can be incorporated into a comprehensive systemwide QA plan.

In trauma systems, guidelines for QA written by the ACEP[19] have emphasized the difference between facility-based and system-based QA. In this trauma model, facility-based QA evaluates the care of individual patients at specific trauma centers, whereas system-based QA examines the overall functioning of the system. For example, system-based QA would include examination of system access, triage protocols, prehospital care, deaths, interhospital transfer, rehabilitation, etc. This approach emphasizes the importance of time from the initial point of injury in the field through the final phase of rehabilitation.

This concept of facility-based QA versus system-based QA for trauma systems can be expanded to complete EMS systems as component-based versus system-based QA. Component-based QA plans would focus on individual system components, such as dispatch centers, BLS services, ALS ground and air services, medical command centers, and receiving facilities. System-based QA plans, on the other hand, would focus on the integration of the components into a system of patient care. In addition a system-based plan should supervise, coordinate, and direct the QA activities of the system components.

In most EMS systems, QA plans are written based on QA done within individual components, with no system-based coordination and supervision. This occurs simply because it is difficult to do systemwide analysis of patient care and easy to focus exclusively on one component, such as one ambulance service. With individual components, data collection is easier, data analysis and feedback of results are less threatening and more private, and concerns regarding legal discoverability are less pressing. Conversely, data collection from several components within a system may be more difficult logistically and may involve more complicated legal issues involving questions of protection discoverability.

Development of a Systemwide Quality Assurance Program

System Structure

It is important to address structure separately from content when developing systemwide QA programs. This must be done for a number of practical and theoretical reasons. Organizing the structure of the program before the content of the program is written serves to encourage participation at all levels and foster cooperation between different components of the system. Proper structure allows providers from many different areas to be involved in writing the program from the very start, which can improve the credibility and effectiveness of the program. It further permits the plan to be dynamic, allowing widespread evaluation and update of the plan. Proper structure can also avoid the unhappy situation in which a large, complicated, and detailed QA plan established by state EMS agency proves to be unusable because of local cost or labor issues.

The structure of a systemwide QA program involves three general layers: the central lead agency, the peripheral system components and providers, and levels of tiers of oversight layered between the center and the periphery. Each agency in these layers should act through a formal committee to coordinate QA activities. This means that every agency, component, and provider has active input into the QA system.

Lead Agency's Role

In building a systemwide structure for QA, the central lead agency has the ultimate responsibility for oversight. It must provide direction while avoiding the pitfalls of a plan that is too bureaucratic, too centralized, or too distant from the neighborhoods where care is actually rendered. The lead agency must be able to ask important questions about patient care. These questions may be difficult to answer and may cross multiple political and economic lines involving several different system components. These components must work together to look at patient-care issues and be responsible for providing answers. An example of a central lead agency is a state EMS agency. A statewide EMS QA committee would be charged with ultimate oversight responsibility and should communicate with successively peripheral committees.

Peripheral Components' Roles

The most peripheral system components and care providers must be included. An ideal systemwide program would include all the 14 or 15 components enumerated previously. An example of a less comprehensive list would still include dispatching centers, BLS services, ALS ground and air services, EMS receiving facilities, and medical command facilities. Each of these system components should have a QA committee that would be responsible for activities within that specific component and would report to local, regional, or central EMS agencies.

Levels of Oversight

Between the central lead agency and the peripheral system components, several levels or tiers of oversight should be layered. Examples of such tiers are local or regional EMS agencies, which would work closely with the local system components and providers and then report to the state EMS agency. These local or regional EMS committees would provide tiers of oversight and create levels of graded responsibility to supervise individual services or components. These local or regional EMS QA committees should then report to the state EMS committee and facilitate meaningful dialogue between the center and the periphery of the system. With this structure the local, regional, and state agencies function primarily to oversee the QA process and to help identify trends. The actual data collection, analysis, and reporting are the responsibility of the individual components or services, although they can use the local and regional EMS agencies as resources.

   In this structure, QA activities can be integrated throughout the system from the periphery to the center. QA activities must flow from individual BLS and

ALS services, through local and regional EMS agencies, into the EMS lead agency, and then back from the center to the periphery. This structure allows dialogue that can identify appropriate issues for systemwide improvement.

Pitfalls in EMS Quality Assurance Plans

There are several pitfalls to be avoided in designing EMS QA programs. Some of these pitfalls are common to QA plans in general, some are common to EMS plans in particular, and some are specific to large EMS systemwide plans. The size of the EMS system is usually directly proportional to the difficulty of meaningful systemwide QI; the bigger the system, the more difficult it is to effect QI.

The QA plan must be patient-care oriented and must avoid "bean counting." It is most important to ask the right questions and avoid collecting meaningless data. Data should be collected only if they can be subjected to analysis that will provide significant and timely feedback on actual patient care. In large systems or systemwide plans much effort, time, and cost can be wasted collecting data that are never used. This generates reluctance to do the work of data collection and loss of credibility for the entire process. It is important to monitor a certain amount of paperwork details, such as the requirement that all trip reports must be complete; however, the ultimate purpose of QI clearly should be to improve patient care. Nothing should be required that does not impact the evaluation of patient care, and data unrelated to improving patient care should not be considered.

The QA program must focus on the periphery, where patient care is actually delivered. In systemwide programs or even large program components such as a large ambulance service, QA tends to be too centralized. QI does not occur in the headquarters of an EMS system or in a QA office somewhere, although the providers may perceive QA in this fashion. Participation from the providers is the only way to get timely and meaningful feedback to improve actual patient care. When data are collected centrally throughout a system, it often takes too long to assemble and analyze them. By the time results are available the information is outdated, the providers have changed, or the system itself has changed.

The QA program must be as participatory as possible. Ideally, a critical mass of people providing care should be involved in the QA planning from the very beginning. This means participation should occur from the initial stages of designing the program's structure and content all the way through implementation of the program. The initial step to encourage participation is to educate providers in the modern principles of CQI. QA that originates from one office does not encourage people to participate in a process in which improved patient care should be a continuous goal.

The program emphasis must be perceived as producing improvement, not as being punitive. Although events must be monitored and sometimes investigated for specific problems, the emphasis should be on trends to produce significant improvement of the system.

Content of a Systemwide Quality Assurance Program

The content of a systemwide QA plan should be flexible and responsive to changes for continuous improvement of the system. This can be accomplished if the QA program is properly structured. Examples of the content of a systemwide QA program will be presented in succeeding chapters. Issues that cross geopolitical boundaries (e.g., field-trauma triage, air-ambulance use, regional dispatch) should be a part of systemwide review. Items that require large databases and complex analyses (e.g., cardiac arrest and trauma registries) should also be system based. Most other components should be reviewed at the periphery, where data and feedback can be given most efficiently. Program content must be dictated by local needs, circumstances, and available resources.

Summary

QA programs for EMS systems can be designed to be meaningful to providers and to improve patient care if several important principles are understood and implemented. EMS system programs should integrate the QI activities of EMS components within a systemwide structure to foster participation and flexibility. Both component- and system-based QI issues should be incorporated. The relatively new principles of CQI are particularly well suited to EMS systems and should be integrated into EMS quality programs. The more traditional QA guidelines of Donabedian, the JCAHO, and the AMA can be used in EMS QA. The focus, however, should be on system processes rather than individuals, on trends rather than individual occurrences, and on education rather than sanctions.

REFERENCES

1. AMA Council of Medical Service: Guidelines for quality assurance, *JAMA* 259:2572-2573, 1988.
2. Association of Air Medical Services (AAMS) Quality Assurance Committee: AAMS resource document for air medical quality assurance programs, *J Air Med Transport* 23-26, 1990.
3. Berwick DM: Continuous improvement as an ideal in health care, *N Engl J Med* 320:53-56, 1989.
4. Crosby P: *Quality without tears: the art of hassle-free management,* New York, 1984, McGraw-Hill, Inc.
5. Deming WE: *Out of the crisis,* Cambridge, Mass, 1982, Massachusetts Institute of Technology, Center for Advanced Engineering Study.
6. Donabedian A: Promoting quality through evaluating the process of patient care, *Med Care* 6:181-202, 1968.
7. Donabedian A: The quality of care: how can it be assessed? *JAMA* 260:1743-1748, 1988.
8. Eastes L, Jacobsen J, editors: *Quality assurance in air medical transport,* Orem, Utah, 1990, WordPerfect Publishing Co.

9. Eisenberg M et al: Cardiac arrest and resuscitation: a tale of 29 cities, *Ann Emerg Med* 19:179-186, 1990.
10. Eisenberg M et al: Out of hospital cardiac arrest: review of the major studies and a proposed uniform reporting system, *Am J Public Health* 70:236-240, 1980.
11. Eitel D et al: Out of hospital cardiac arrest: a six year experience in a suburban-rural system, *Ann Emerg Med* 17:808-812, 1988.
12. Gray C, Kaiser K: *Examples of monitoring and evaluation in emergency services,* Chicago, 1988, Joint Commission on Accreditation of Healthcare Organizations.
13. Holroyd BR, Knopp R, Kollsen G: Medical control: quality assurance in prehospital care, *JAMA* 256(8):1027-1021, 1986.
14. Holroyd B et al: Prehospital patients refusing care, *Ann Emerg Med* 17:957-963, 1988.
15. Kuehl A, editor: *National association of EMS physicians EMS medical directors' handbook,* St. Louis, 1989, Mosby–Year Book.
16. Newman M: Comparing apples with apples: time for a standard definition of survival from out-of-hospital cardiac arrest, *American Heart Association and Citizen CPR Foundation Newsletter: Currents in Emergency Cardiac Care* 1:2-3, 1990.
17. Pennsylvania Department of Health, Division of Emergency Medical Services: Protocols for prehospital triage and interhospital transfer of trauma patients, Harrisburg, Pa, January 1990, The Department.
18. Roush WR, McDowell RM: *Emergency medical services systems.* In Roush WR, editor: *Principles of EMS systems: a comprehensive text for physicians,* Dallas, 1989, American College of Emergency Physicians.
19. American College of Emergency Physicians: *Trauma care systems quality assurance guidelines.* In: *Guidelines for trauma care systems,* March 1990, The College.
20. Walton M: *The Deming management method,* New York, 1986, Putnam Publishing Group.
21. Berwick DM, Godfrey AB, Roessner J: *Curing health care: new strategies for quality improvement,* San Francisco, 1990, Jossey-Bass Inc, Publishers.
22. Kritchevsky SB, Simmons BP: Continuous quality improvement: concepts and applications for physician care, *JAMA* 266(13):1817-1823, 1991.

3

Developing Standards for EMS Quality Improvement

Alexander Kuehl, M.D.

Identifying local levels of performance that are considered acceptable by a recognized authority to evaluate EMS activities is critical to the adequate functioning of all EMS systems. These identified levels of performance are commonly called standards or norms, and they facilitate the successful structuring of an ongoing quality improvement (QI) mechanism.

Standards can be developed for virtually any objective EMS activity, including areas as diverse as personnel physical requirements, cognitive and psychomotor success in education, ambulance response time, vehicle maintenance, medical supplies and equipment availability, and actual medical treatment. There are also subjective aspects of EMS for which it is more difficult to develop standards; these often deal with interpersonal issues, such as the patient's satisfaction with the prehospital care.

History

After the evacuation of Dunkirk in 1940, the British Home Guard trained to repel the impending German invasion. One story tells of a young officer given command of a local artillery unit made up of six rather elderly men, all veterans of the Great War. Each time the gun crew unlimbered the artillery piece from the truck, only four of the men would actually operate the gun; the other two would stand at attention near the truck. The young officer was confused and frustrated because no one could explain the job of the "extra" two men. Finally, a very old man, a veteran of the Boer War, explained that they were "holding the horses." This is an example of a standard that was once relevant; it had become outdated yet still lived on.

It is interesting to note that major federal initiatives regarding both EMS and medical quality assurance (QA) (now QI) began as parts of President Richard M. Nixon's legislative health package in the early 1970s. No one then could have imagined the results that those programs would ultimately deliver. In the early days of the Professional Standards Review Organization (PSRO) initiative the major battles were over both the nature of the standards to be created and the person to develop those standards. It was quickly learned that although standards could be developed *de novo,* they needed to evolve gradually to be accepted in a national environment.

Need for Consensus

Standards should never simply be copied from a reference book; rather, standards are best developed through consensus building. Although there are undoubtedly EMS system directors, chiefs of operation, and medical directors who have the wisdom and the administrative authority to independently develop and implement new standards, the better political course is to fully involve as many individuals and organizations as possible in the process. Without such involvement there cannot be consensus, and without consensus, it is all but impossible to implement a standard, especially if no specific legislative or regulatory authority exists. Standards are much too fragile to survive without consensus. This axiom applies not only when developing medical care standards, such as advanced life support treatment protocols, but also when developing standards for equipment, personnel, and administrative operations. It is appropriate for the EMS system field providers to participate in the development of institutional standards for the hospitals operating within the EMS system; however, the inpatient experts should obviously take the lead.

In New York City, standards and the resulting protocols were developed for the triage of patients at the scene so that some patients could be safely selected not to be transported to a hospital. It was clear to the supervising EMS medical director that patients were routinely being informally and dangerously triaged by prehospital providers throughout the city; therefore, an attempt was made to formalize that process by requiring consultation with direct medical control physicians. Although similar procedures existed in other jurisdictions a political battle ensued in New York City, ultimately leading to a great deal of bitterness among medical control physicians and physician members of the city administration.

The main but unstated reason for New York City's crisis was that the general medical community had not been asked for meaningful input prior to the initial protocol and standard development. The stated reason for resistance was concern that sick patients would be left at the scene, and therefore the protocol was encumbered with layers of clinical reviews and redundancies. When behind-the-scenes negotiations were unable to resolve this conflict, the EMS medical director was obliged to carry out the program in the face of intense criticism from the medical community. Of course, this undermined the authority of the medical director and gave the wrong message to the providers in the field. Years later there is still no meaningful process for denying transport from the scene. In summary, the standard-making process must be a cooperative process; if important players do not have access to the process, they will be in a position to torpedo most medical and operational recommendations.

Timing

A given EMS system should be neither the first nor the last to develop and implement standards concerning a given topic. The logic of such an attitude should be clear; the innovative EMS system that first introduces a new set of operational standards will often be bogged down by either defending those new standards or correcting the glitches. Of course the system that waits and is last to introduce new standards will spend months or even years languishing unnecessarily in a suboptimal situation.

Geographic Standards

EMS standards may be developed locally, regionally, at the state level, or nationally. Yet the implications and the processes are different at each of those levels. For example, local standards rarely have the force of law, yet they are often universally accepted and followed if there was broad-based consensus during the developmental phase. Regional standards are often weak since few regional bodies are capable of enforcing such standards; also at a regional level, broad-based consensus is almost impossible to obtain. State-level standards are generally very powerful, but they may be highly unpopular, usually because they have the legal force of rule, regulation, or even law. For most ambulance providers the state is the most significant regulating force; therefore state-developed standards are often the strongest and the most useful for a local QI program.

National standards promulgated by the federal government are generally very powerful, although national standards developed by voluntary organizations, such as the American Society for Testing and Materials (ASTM),[1,11] are relatively easily sidestepped. The national standards of nongovernmental groups may be ignored. When voluntary standards become a formal part of a certification program, they develop power. Occasionally legislators will be asked to write specific organizational suggestions into law as standards (e.g., the American Heart Association Advanced Cardiac Life Support training); thoughtful legislators are generally careful to ensure that standards written into law remain generic. Certification and accreditation are effective means of implementing standards on a national level. Several efforts are currently under way to certify or accredit ambulance services.

The newly formed Commission on Accreditation of Ambulance Services (CAAS) is a multidisciplinary body composed of physicians, nurses, fire chiefs, and state EMS directors. It has developed very detailed standards in excess of national minimums to serve as a "gold standard" for ambulance services. This process will serve as a means for EMS organizations to distinguish themselves as quality organizations and may confer a marketing advantage or a possible advantage for reimbursement in the future.[8]

Similarly the Joint Review Committee on Educational Programs for Emergency Medical Technician-Paramedics is a national organization that reviews and certifies paramedic training programs. This process is also not mandatory for paramedic training but serves to distinguish those programs certified as meeting a higher level of excellence. Although not forcing change, standards that are perceived to connote excellence will continue to generate interest and efforts to comply with them.

Internal Considerations

Introducing and adopting standards forces change, and change is usually painful. When change is necessary, it is helpful to make as many simultaneous changes as possible. The period of change should be followed by a period of stability and integration. Middle-level managers often garble—intentionally or otherwise—administrative messages that initiate or explain change. This happens either because those managers do not want to take "heat" from the employees or because they do not agree with the proposed changes.

James Page, an EMS philosopher, occasionally speaks about the universal existence of negatively oriented mid-level managers who, although bright, have been passed over for leadership and who consequently resist change by any new management team. These individuals must be reckoned with and their biases neutralized before meaningful change is possible in an organization. Often, there is a tendency to attempt to circumvent such individuals; however, they should be dealt with directly. Reticent middle managers must become involved in the process for it to succeed. Traditionally they are circumvented by adding another layer of bureaucracy to replace the dysfunctional layer. Nowadays, however, simply adding an additional layer of bureaucracy to perform their function is just too expensive. For that economic reason, if for no other, such resistance to change must be approached directly and cooperation obtained if at all possible.

External Considerations

Other players in the EMS game may fear that implementing a new standard will produce changes. In 1987 the medical director of New York City EMS proposed a standard requiring that all cardiac arrests have a response time of less than 6 minutes instead of the previous 10-minute average for all life-threatening calls. But when the city's mayor discovered that the proportion of cardiac-arrest calls answered in less than 6 minutes was only about 50%, he immediately vetoed the new standard. Concern was raised that ambulances would not meet the standard half the time. The city's financial people, who were sure that the new standard would require many more ambulances, sighed in relief. In reality, though, by simply changing the way the existing ambulances were dispatched to "cat-bite calls," New York City EMS could have met the standard and saved an additional 100 lives per year.

Implementing Standards

Once standards are developed and approved they must be explained and implemented in a relatively easy manner to understand directive or protocol. Following a period of education and questioning the standards must be rigorously enforced. One of the greatest political liabilities that an EMS leader can assume is to have developed and promulgated standards that are either not enforced or, worse yet, are not enforceable.

For example, during the mid-1980s, many EMS systems began to require field units to notify direct medical control when patients refused to go to the hospital. These notifications were made mandatory in response to a number of untoward outcomes in which patients were left at home, only to later develop severe medical complications. Although it was important to deal with such a problem, this simple across-the-board standard overloaded the medical control capabilities of urban systems. Although the standards and the resulting protocols were medically appropriate and reasonable, they were simply too much trouble to be enforced by middle-level management. Very quickly, field units recognized that such notifications were effectively not required. The behavior of field personnel returned to the prestandard situation, but now the system had become vulnerable since it was liable for not enforcing its own standards.

Subjective Standards Are Objective Problems

There are some prehospital activities for which it is difficult, if not impossible, to develop standards. In the previously cited example involving an EMS system's refusal to transport inappropriate patients, there were two difficulties: (1) trying to encourage prehospital providers to initiate a process that would decrease their workload *and* (2) requiring them to formally access medical control if they questioned whether a patient needed to be transported. The prehospital providers were to simply report their objective findings to medical control; however, personnel felt at risk initiating a formal process based on their own evaluation. Previously they were comfortable with their subjective but informal on-the-scene decisions to leave patients; however, when the prehospital providers were held accountable, such decisions became uncomfortable.

Craft Standards Carefully

Standards need to be tailored to individual systems. For example, early in the 1980s trauma center standards were most often developed individually by each locality. As a consequence the process was relatively straightforward until hospitals recognized that there might be limited numbers of designated trauma centers. The process then became political.

Unfortunately the designation process became even more confused when the American College of Surgeons (ACS) introduced the so-called level 1, level 2, and level 3 designations for trauma centers with defined national guidelines for each. These guidelines became national standards, and many systems used them without first considering the type of trauma system actually required by the local jurisdiction and without first allowing local experts to modify them. In New Jersey, where the standards were developed locally through a consensus mechanism, the process of statewide trauma center development progressed smoothly; in Pennsylvania, which rigidly adhered to the ACS methodology, the designation process was aborted on several occasions before being modified for local use.

In New York City, trauma center standards were approved in the early 1980s for only one level (an amalgam of ACS level 1 and level 2). Had the ACS standards been used the city would have been left with four or five level-1 trauma centers (mostly in Manhattan) and dozens of level-2 trauma centers spread across the remainder of the city. What the city needed was 12 or 14 well-distributed trauma centers, which in fact is what the locally modified process ultimately provided. Unfortunately, as trauma center designation continues at the New York State level, the standard-making process once again resembles the ACS model, and almost every hospital may be some sort of a trauma center. Therefore it is possible that many level-2 and level-3 trauma centers meeting a new set of state standards may emerge and destroy the currently functioning system.

Standards May Differ in Philosophy

Standards may be developed in any number of different philosophic fashions. A standard may be a baseline or minimal goal that absolutely must be met for that specific aspect of the EMS system to be acceptable; it may be an optimal achievable goal that is, in effect, a standard both obtainable and satisfactory; or it may be a goal that is set intentionally high so as to stimulate either efforts by the participants to excel or funding by the budget director. Unachievable standards are dangerous from a medical-legal standpoint since such standards effectively create lightning rods for criticism and litigation. It is important, but very difficult, to explain to well-meaning emergency physicians and others why optimal but economically unachievable standards are a problem for EMS medical directors to implement, especially in financially strapped municipalities.

Summary

Compliance with standards and comparison with performance parameters are no longer the sole effective measures of quality in an EMS system. Today the ultimate goal is improvement; that is, we must capture information about each prehospital interaction, integrate that information into conclusions that improve system performance, and then share that information with the public. The standards developed by the system will usually act as both the daily operational targets *and* the measuring devices for system evaluation. Those standards must be crafted deliberately and with vision; otherwise they may become irrelevant, or worse, guide the system in unintended directions.

REFERENCES

1. American Society for Testing and Materials: *Annual book of ASTM standards,* vol 13.01, Philadelphia, 1988, The Society.
2. American College of Surgeons: *Bull Am Coll Surg* 64:43-48, Chicago, 1979.
3. Codman EA: The product of a hospital, *Surg Gynecol Obstet* 1914:118.
4. Deming WE: *Out of the crisis,* Cambridge, 1986, Massachusetts Institute of Technology Press.
5. Donabedian A: The quality of medical care, *Science* 200:1856-1884, 1978.
6. National Association of EMS Physicians: *Emergency medical dispatching,* Pittsburgh, 1987, The Association.
7. Johnson JC: *Quality assurance in EMS.* In Roush WR, editor: *Principles of EMS systems,* Dallas, 1989, American College of Emergency Physicians.
8. Page JO: CAAS: A new gold standard, *JEMS* 6, 1991.
9. American Hospital Association: *Provisional Guidelines for Optional Categorization of Hospital Emergency Capabilities,* Chicago, 1981, The Association.
10. Ryan J: *Quality assurance.* In Kuehl AE, (editor:) The NAEMSP medical directors handbook, St. Louis, 1989, Mosby—Year Book.
11. American Society for Testing and Materials: *Standard practice for qualifications, responsibilities and authority of individuals and institutions providing medical direction of emergency medical services,* Philadelphia, 1988, The Society.
12. Thompson R: Some practical applications of Deming's points, *J Qual Assur* pp 22-23, 1990.

4

Evaluation of System Components

James Pointer, M.D.

Evaluation of the emergency medical services (EMS) system and its components constitutes the analytical portion of the quality assurance (QA) process. Once standards have been developed, assessing them is the next logical step. This chapter reviews the methods for evaluating a number of EMS system components. The medical control hospital audit method of evaluation both summarizes the chapter's concepts and provides a practical example for EMS system managers.

Evaluation of the System

An overall assessment of the EMS system is necessary before evaluation of the quality of its individual components. The list of EMS components in the EMS act of 1973 is still useful to identify EMS system components (see Chapter 2).

In a sense these system components are the essential overall structural standards for a good EMS system; each component must be present. However, the list is too broad to set standards for QA. Instead, EMS managers must develop standards for these system components based on established or community norms.

Access and dispatch are included in this section because they are prerequisites for a quality EMS system.

Desirable structural standards for EMS system access are shown in the box on page 37. Rapid consumer access to 9-1-1 and the expeditious triage of appropriate calls to medical dispatch are critical. Rapid response times and state-of-the-art patient care are undermined if a system is characterized by long delays in transferring emergency calls to the medical dispatcher.

Desirable Structural Standards and Methods of Evaluating EMS System Access

I. Structural standards

    A. 9-1-1 in place
    B. Rapid triage to medical dispatch
    C. Translation services
    D. Poison-control interface

II. Methods of evaluation

    A. Time-interval reports
    B. Consumer questionnaire
    C. Online supervision
    D. Audit

Evaluating patient access to EMS is often problematic. Emergency number public safety answering points (PSAPs) are often managed by public service agencies over which EMS or local medical control has no jurisdiction. Allocation of 9-1-1 operations may have more to do with police department funding or community crime statistics than with medical need. Close coordination among jurisdictional agencies and enabling legislation for those agencies are crucial. Methods of evaluating EMS system access are also set forth in the box shown above.

As with other system components, online supervision is most effective in evaluating the process. For example, written documentation and the use of a "script" for callers are important process standards for measuring access. Online supervision is the best method for ensuring timely and accurate compliance with these standards. Computer-generated reports are often used as important or sole QA methods. Sample reports include a listing of basic life support (BLS) calls subsequently upgraded to advanced life support (ALS) or all cases transported as emergencies. These tools can assess the accuracy of priority dispatch.[2,5]

Audits can also be a cost-effective, productive, and thorough method of evaluation. The technique is applicable to every EMS system component, but it must be carefully planned and conducted. Independent, expert, impartial evaluators are the best auditors. Of course a formal audit employing such auditors may be expensive. The planning of a medical control hospital audit is reviewed in detail later in this chapter.

Desirable EMS system dispatch standards and methods of evaluation are listed in the box on page 38. Physician and dispatcher supervision are necessary in the dispatch center to monitor medical and procedural processes. *Dispatch data* refer to time-milestone information that is usually collected through computer-aided dispatch (CAD) systems. Although this information evaluates the time necessary for dispatch and field activities, it is almost always collected at the

---

Desirable Structural Standards and Methods of Evaluation for EMS System Dispatch

I. Structural standards

   A. Dispatch priority algorithms/protocols
   B. Prearrival telephone instructions
   C. Medical control of algorithms/protocols
   D. QA plan

II. Methods of evaluation

   A. Online supervision
     1. Medical
     2. Dispatcher
   B. Tape reviews
   C. Feedback reports
   D. Dispatch and field data

---

dispatch center. EMS managers, consumers, and politicians often place exaggerated importance on several of the EMS dispatch and field-time intervals.

Figure 4-1 provides these intervals and milestones. First, however, a few definitions are in order. *Determine time* is the period of time a dispatcher takes to determine the appropriate ambulance response (e.g., code II or code III, ALS or BLS, urgent or emergent, hot or cold); it is the interval between the time the call is determined and the time the ambulance is dispatched. *Queue time* is the period of time a caller waits for an available ambulance, the interval between when the call is received and when the call is determined. For example, queue time will be

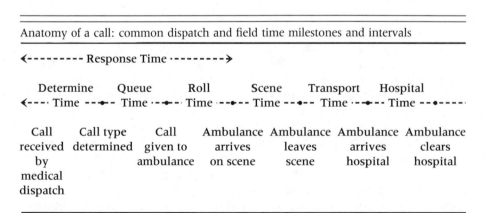

Anatomy of a call: common dispatch and field time milestones and intervals

Figure 4-1 EMS managers must establish consistent terminology and reasonable standards for dispatch.

Table 4-1. Ideal Dispatch and Field Interval Standards

Time interval	Ideal time
Determine time	<30 sec, 90th percentile
Queue time	0
Roll time	5 min, 90th percentile
Response time	<8 min, 90th percentile
Field time	<20 min
Transport time	
Urban	<10 min
Rural	<30 min
Hospital time	<15 min

zero if an ambulance is immediately available. *Roll time* is the interval between the time of dispatch of the ambulance and arrival on the scene. *Response time,* strictly speaking, is the determine time, queue time, and roll time added together. It is the interval between receipt of the call by the medical dispatcher and arrival of the ambulance on the scene.

These intervals, particularly response time, are emphasized because of the attention they receive in the medical literature and often the press. EMS planners need to establish consistent definitions and ideal outcome standards for these intervals. Although there are no validated dispatch-interval standards in the EMS literature, suggested time-interval standards based on those used by jurisdictions throughout the United States are presented in Table 4-1.

Evaluation of System Components

First Responders and EMT-Basics

Even though first responders and basic emergency medical technicians (EMTs) provide initial and often life-saving care, these providers are often omitted from the QA plan. Although paramedics may be overregulated by the authorizing agency and overscrutinized by medical control, first responders and EMTs are often free of medical control and formal policy and procedure. For example, California has lengthy state and local policies governing paramedics. For first responders and EMTs the state's regulations cover only early defibrillation.

Listed in the box on page 40 are structural standards and methods for evaluating first responders and EMTs. Both medical and procedural policies are necessary; policies that pertain to interaction with transporting agencies are particularly important. Early defibrillation capability and basic EMT training have become the standard of care in many urban and rural areas. First responders and EMTs should be qualified to perform scene triage in a two-tiered system even if triage is performed by dispatch. Some triage provides a check on dispatch triage and helps prevent "undertriage." Finally, first responders and

---

Desirable Structural Standards and Methods of Evaluation for First Responders and EMT-Basics

I. Structural standards

  A. Written protocols
    1. Medical
    2. Procedural
  B. Level of training $\geq$ basic EMT
  C. Early defibrillation capability
  D. Scene triage (two-tiered systems)
  E. Medical control and QA plan

II. Methods of evaluation

  A. Response times and other intervals
  B. Online supervision
  C. Online medical control
  D. Peer review (retrospective)
  E. Tape review
  F. Medical control module review
  G. Audits

EMTs, like other prehospital personnel, should complete a written patient encounter form. This provides a relatively simple, though not comprehensive, method of assessing performance.

Several of the methods of evaluation deserve comment. Response times and other intervals are as important for first responders and EMTs as they are for paramedics. The advent of early defibrillation using automatic or semiautomatic devices has magnified the importance of these responders. Although most physicians and providers can identify a number of clinical entities impacted by prehospital care, ventricular fibrillation is the only condition documented in the medical literature to be clearly influenced by prehospital personnel. Favorable survival rates associated with early ventricular fibrillation mandate more QA efforts for those who place the paddles to the chest. Most defibrillator manufacturers provide a medical control module in their machines. EMS system managers should choose automatic and semiautomatic devices that offer this module, which greatly facilitates QA.

Paramedics

Paramedic services are the backbone of most EMS systems. Paramedic response times and other field intervals often factor prominently in contracts between paramedic providers and EMS political jurisdictions. In the large majority of EMS systems there are simply insufficient resources to respond to each call as rapidly as desired. In the 1990s and beyond, it is mandatory to earmark resources for patients who truly need paramedic service to save life and preserve limb. Thus EMS managers must expend more effort (and research dollars) to distinguish the calls for which rapid response times are truly essential.

Paramedics provide all the emergent care in the majority of systems. In spite of the wide variety of system configurations and the diversity of medical control, paramedics are generally subject to more regulation and QA than other system components. Paramedic QA must cover three broad areas of prehospital care: assessment, treatment, and skills maintenance. Because assessment and treatment may occur simultaneously, EMS managers should evaluate these areas together for QA purposes.[6]

Comparing paramedic field assessments with emergency department diagnoses can be a valuable outcome standard. To accomplish this, one must categorize both assessments and diagnoses into broad but distinct groups. Some researchers divide categories along "system" lines (e.g., cardiovascular). A comparison may then be done using computers.

System managers can develop process standards and criteria for a wide range of paramedic activities. Written documentation and tape-recorded paramedic runs can be checked against these criteria. Regular reports that specify deficiencies and follow trends may be developed for each provider and each paramedic.[15] To ensure consistency in clinical assessments EMS managers can compare paramedic clinical assessment data with those of nurses,[1] physicians, or paramedic supervisors. A comparison can be performed simultaneously on the same patient and the results documented for QA purposes. Medical control officers can also use a review of unanticipated therapies as an outcome standard. This method, also highly adaptable to computer spread-sheet or database software, highlights unusual or unexpected paramedic treatment modalities for a studied patient condition.[4]

The box on page 42 gives structural standards for evaluation of paramedics, methods for evaluating paramedic patient assessment and treatment, and methods of evaluating skills maintenance. It is difficult to prioritize the importance of these methods of evaluation. Methods used depend strongly on local resources, system configuration, and needs. However, comparison of paramedic field assessment with emergency department (ED) diagnosis should be at the top of the system manager's QA list.

Receiving Hospitals

The receiving hospital is a critical EMS system component. Unfortunately, it may be difficult to set standards for or incorporate receiving hospitals into the QA plan. Often, *tradeoff* (the sharing of system data and training resources) is necessary to ensure participation of a receiving facility. For example, receiving hospitals may be quite willing to provide outcome information on admitted patients if, in return, these hospitals are provided system demographic and destination statistics. (Obviously, the promulgation of these standards may be subject to considerable politics.)

Desirable Structural Standards and Evaluation Methods for Paramedics

I. Structural standards

  A. Prescribed equipment
  B. Written protocols
    1. Medical
    2. Provider interface
    3. Destination
      a. Response times and other intervals
  C. Medical control and QA plan

II. Methods of evaluation—patient assessment and treatment

  A. Online supervision
    1. Online medical control[3]
    2. Comparison with emergency department/hospital diagnosis[13]
    3. Documentation—explicit versus implicit criteria[16]
      a. Computer-assisted audits[15]
    4. Peer review
    5. Concurrent radio skill review
  B. Tape review
  C. Comparison of clinical data elements with those performed by nurses/physicians[1]
    1. Outcome
      a. Survival
      b. Length of stay
    2. Review of unanticipated therapies[4]
    3. Audits

III. Methods of evaluation—skills maintenance[7]

  A. Online supervision
  B. Physician verification[11]
  C. Success rates
  D. Outcome
  E. Audits

Because the EMS system manager often has no authority to mandate receiving-hospital standards, it may be necessary to tie compliance to the delivery of ambulance patients. The care rendered the patient by the receiving hospital is quite important. An excellent dispatch system, 3-minute response times, early defibrillation, appropriate assessment and treatment, and quick transport times may prove inadequate if the receiving hospital does not perform satisfactorily. The box on page 43 provides the structural, process, and outcome standards, as well as the major methods of evaluation, for receiving hospitals.

Desirable Structural, Process and Outcome Standards, and Evaluation Methods for Receiving Hospitals

I. Structural standards

  A. Recordkeeping
  B. Personnel
    1. Physicians
      a. Board certificate
      b. Special certifications (e.g., pediatric advanced life support)
      c. Resident coverage
    2. Nurses
      a. Certification
      b. Continuing education (CE)
  C. Services and equipment
    1. Referral and transfer agreements
    2. Medical equipment
    3. Communication equipment

II. Process standards

  A. Compliance with laws, regulations
  B. EMS committee activity
  C. Data collection and analysis
  D. Provision of orientation, training, and CE in EMS
  E. Participation in EMS QA
  F. Participation in disaster planning
  G. Acceptance of all patients

III. Outcome standards

  A. Outcome data
    1. Survival
    2. Length of stay
    3. Other
  B. Passing score on audit

IV. Evaluation methods

  A. Paramedic feedback
  B. Self-assessment tool
  C. Audits
  D. Patient-satisfaction surveys

Because of the usually noncontractual nature of the relationship between the receiving hospital and the authorizing or medical control agency, the self-assessment tool may be the most viable method for evaluating QA standards. This procedure allows the hospital to grade itself using standards provided by the community or the authorizing agency. This document may be used by the

Desirable Structural, Process and Outcome Standards for Medical Control Hospitals

I. Structural standards

A. Recordkeeping
B. Personnel
C. Physicians (including medical director, medical control nurses, and paramedics)
  1. Board certification
  2. Special certifications
  3. Minimum full-time equivalents
D. Services and equipment (meet or exceed receiving-hospital standards)
  1. Clerical support
  2. Computer hardware and software
  3. Adequate office space
  4. Supplies for exchange
  5. Redundant communication equipment
  6. Recording equipment

II. Process standards

A. Compliance with laws, regulations
B. Committee membership
C. Documentation, data collection, and analysis
D. Training, orientation, and CE in EMS issues
E. Participation in system QA
F. Participation in disaster planning
G. Participation in prehospital research
H. Online medical control
  1. Physician, medical control nurse/paramedic, and staffing
  2. Duties and responsibilities
I. Field observation for physicians and medical control nurses
J. CE requirements for physicians and medical control nurses

III. Outcome standards

A. Outcome
  1. Survival
  2. Length of stay
  3. Other
B. Audit performance[12]
C. Response time to medical control radio

Selected Medical Control Hospital QA Goals
Personnel

---

1. Physicians
   - American Board of Emergency Medicine certification
   - Expertise/certification in pediatrics, trauma, cardiac-life support
   - 12 hours per year in paramedic CE/teaching
   - 24 hours per year field observation
   - 30 second, at 90th percentile, response time to medical control radio
2. Medical control nurses
   - Critical care or emergency certification
   - Expertise/certification in pediatrics, trauma, cardiac-life support
   - 12 hours per year in paramedic CE/teaching
   - 24 hours per year field observation
   - Dedicated staffing (2 dedicated nurses if > 3.5 calls per hour)
   - 15 second, at 90th percentile, response time to medical control radio
3. Clerical support—0.5 FTE per 20,000 calls
4. Data collection and analysis
5. Computer hardware and database program with linkage to receiving hospital and authorizing agency
6. Regular process and outcome reports

---

hospital for evaluation and planning or by the medical control agency in lieu of a site visit or another more formal method of evaluation.

Medical Control Hospitals

Most EMS systems use one or more hospitals to provide medical control. This control usually includes online medical direction by physicians, nurses, and/or paramedics. Because this facility acts as a medical control surrogate of the authorizing agency, there should be a formal agreement or contract between that authorizing agency and medical control hospital. Even in systems in which the authorizing agency and the medical control hospital are one and the same, there are usually QA standards imposed by the county, region, or state.

Medical control hospitals are often totally responsible for system QA. These facilities must play an integral, if not lead, role in EMS QA. The box on page 44 gives standards for use in medical control hospitals. The box above presents specific goals for various medical control hospital QA standards.

The Ideal System

The ideal EMS system, from a QA standpoint, is one in which managers have developed not only comprehensive QA standards and criteria but also compre-

---

The Ideal System
Evaluation of System Components

---

1. List objectives of evaluation for each system component
2. Develop evaluation tool that meets objectives
   - Consider resources
   - Evaluate structural, process, and outcome standards
   - Check by ensuring that objectives encompass all QA standards
3. Develop process and reporting mechanism

The Ideal System
Using Limited Resources

---

1. The use of a QA model from another successful system will save resources.
2. Division of QA responsibilities among all providers is cost-effective.
3. Audits provide a great deal of information, and the data can be collected retrospectively.
4. Structural standards are easy to check and are usually met.
5. Dispatch- and field-time interval measurements are available and useful.
6. Online supervision is used to measure process standards.
7. Outcome standards allow your system to be compared with others.
8. Self-assessment surveys are the most cost-effective QA tools.

---

hensive methods of evaluation and feedback to frontline personnel. The first box on this page outlines the process for evaluating components within the ideal system. At best, the chosen standards will emulate those used in the continent's most renowned systems. Minimally, the standards will reflect the best system possible considering available resources. Similarly, the evaluation methods used are dependent on fiscal considerations. The second box on this page summarizes a basic strategy for allocating limited resources in EMS QA. Like the standards it encompasses, the QA process is as important as the QA outcome.

Summary

The focus of this chapter has been the evaluation of the EMS system and its components. To assist in solidifying the concepts presented here the box on page 47 provides a step-by-step guide to evaluating an essential system component, the medical control hospital.

How to Evaluate a System Component
Medical Control Hospital

Step 1: List objectives of evaluation

1. Compliance with laws and regulations
2. Compliance with contract
3. Compliance with policies and procedures
4. Assessment of medical control
5. Documentation
6. Assessment of recordkeeping and organization
7. Observation of online medical control
8. Discussion of improvement of system

Step 2: Develop evaluation tool that meets objectives (medical control hospital audit)

1. Listing of structural process and outcome QA criteria
2. Objectives should contain all QA standards

Step 3: Develop process and reporting mechanism

1. Entrance interview
2. Separate inspections
3. Group meeting
4. Review of online medical control
5. Exit interview
6. Report

The information presented here does not address all the components that must be evaluated by a system QA plan, nor can it. A QA program must be based, first and foremost, on the issues faced by the individual system being evaluated. Components identified here are important areas to any EMS system and should receive scrutiny. However, no system will use all the methods of evaluation discussed. Careful development and prioritization of the QA plan before evaluation of individual components are of paramount importance to the success of the program.

REFERENCES

1. Cayten CG et al: Assessing the validity of EMS data, *JACEP* 7:390-396, 1978.
2. Curka PA et al: Computed-aided EMS priority dispatch: ability of a computerized triage system to safely spare paramedics from responses not requiring advanced life support, *Ann Emerg Med* 19(abstract):456, 1990.
3. Erder MN, Davidson SJ, Cheney RA: On-line medical command in theory and practice, *Ann Emerg Med* 18:261-268, 1989.

4. Hoffman, JR et al: Does paramedic-base hospital contact result in beneficial deviations from standard prehospital protocols? *West J Med* 153:283-287, 1990.
5. Kallsen G, Nabors MD: The use of priority medical dispatch to distinguish between high and low risk patients, *Ann Emerg Med* 19(abstract):458, 1990.
6. Lieske AM: *Standards: The basis of a quality assurance program.* In Meisenheimer CG, editor: *Quality assurance: a complete guide to effective programs,* Rockville, MD, 1985, Aspen Publishers Inc.
7. McKinney B: Evaluating paramedic performance—who is responsible? *STAT* 2:79-81, 1980.
8. McSwain NE: Medical control—what is it? JACEP 7:114-116, 1978.
9. Nicholls ME: *Terminology in quality assurance.* In Nicholls ME, Wessells VG, editors: *Nursing standards and nursing process,* Wahefield, Mass, 1977, Nursing Resources.
10. Page JR, editor: Medical control of emergency medical services: an overview for emergency physicians, Dallas, 1984, American College of Emergency Physicians.
11. Pointer J: Clinical characteristics of paramedics' performance of endotracheal intubation, *J Emerg Med* 6:505-509, 1988.
12. Pointer J: The advanced life support base hospital audit for medical control in an emergency medical services system, *Ann Emerg Med* 16:577-580, 1987.
13. Pointer JE, Osur MA: Effect of standing orders on field times, *Ann Emerg Med* 18:1119-1121, 1989.
14. Stewart RD: Medical direction in emergency medical services: the role of the physician, Emerg Med Clin North Am 5:99-132, 1987.
15. Swor RA, Hoelzer M: A computer assisted quality assurance audit in a multi-provider EMS system, *Ann Emerg Med* 19:286-290, 1990.
16. Wasserberger J et al: Base station prehospital care: judgement errors and deviations from protocol, *Ann Emerg Med* 16:867-870, 1987.

5

Where to Begin: The Implementation of an Innovation

Ronald G. Pirrallo, M.D.

A plethora of recent texts have promoted the need for change within organizations in the United States.[1,2,7] The terms "total quality management" (TQM) and "continuous quality improvement" (CQI) represent new quality programs. Each philosophy has its own champion and its own followers. Regardless of which program one uses a change must first occur to improve the organization.

This process begins with the implementation of an innovation, which in this context means some device, technique, or concept that is new to the adopting organization.[5] Attempts to explain the change process have been limited by the uniqueness of each innovation and each organization. Ideally, if one could identify the key features of an innovation and an organization, recommendations could then be made for its implementation. Munson and Pelz[6] accomplished this task by developing conditional principles that build a framework to facilitate the change process; in this chapter their principles are applied to an emergency medical services (EMS) system to implement an innovation and improve prehospital care.

This chapter suggests an approach to initiating the change process: the implementation of an innovation. First, a description of the change process and a definition of a successful innovation are proposed. The key features of an innovation and the implementation process (the conditional principles) itself are then discussed. Finally, a method is offered to prepare an EMS organization to accept and preserve the innovation.

Description of the Change Process

The clearest way to conceptualize the change process is to use the classic Lewinian[3] concept of unfreezing, moving, and refreezing. To change, one must first become open to learning *(unfreezing)*. To learn a new technique the provider must be willing to abandon the old technique. Sometimes this step alone can prevent change, which will be discussed in more detail in a later section. The provider can begin to achieve the desired change *(moving)* through education and training. The definitive implementation and survival of an innovation are the goals of the change process *(refreezing)*. The systemwide expansion of a pilot protocol is used as an example. Lewin's intuitive model describes the change process, as well as the potential areas of failure. It is essential to remember, however, that change is a process and not an event.

Defining the Successful Innovation

What does it mean to say that an innovation is a success? The answer may be surprisingly complex. The development of an innovation can be divided into three stages: diagnosis, design, and implementation.[5] At each stage, different criteria can be used to define success, as demonstrated by the following questions:

Diagnosis stage:
- Was an important problem identified and its causes correctly understood?

Design stage:
- Was a solution developed that was both technically sound and compatible with this organization?
- Was the design realistic in terms of organizational resources?

Implementation stage:
- Were the innovation and its procedures thoroughly communicated?
- Was the innovation correctly applied as designed?
- Was the innovation endorsed and supported by all of the essential participants, or actors?
- Did the innovation survive and become incorporated?
- Did the innovation achieve the desired outcomes to improve quality?[5]

Obviously the successful implementation of an innovation requires success in each prior stage. Thus a successful innovation is one that survives and becomes incorporated, resulting in the desired improvement in quality. However, this definition does not guarantee that the content of the incorporated innovation will be the same as that of the original innovation; the implementation process itself can alter the content of an innovation.

Role of the Actors

Every organization is intrinsically political in that ways must be found to create order and direction among people with potentially diverse and conflicting interests.[4] Therefore the change process is influenced not only by the content of the innovation itself, but also by the interests and power of the affected individuals—the participants, or the actors. This is particularly true in EMS systems. Any medical director who has tried to limit a provider's scope of practice is keenly aware of this fact. Unfortunately for an innovation's designers, the actors determine their own interests. Disinterest in change can be as formidable an obstacle as opposition to change. In addition, the power of the actors will vary with the content of each innovation. According to Munson and Pelz[6]:

> The degree of congruence versus conflict among actors' interests in this innovation, and the degree to which their power is diffused versus concentrated, will determine what kind of intervention strategy is required for success.

Building on this statement, several conditional principles can be used to direct the implementation process (Figure 5-1)[6]:

1. When power is concentrated in a small group, such as top management, it is possible for that group to dominate the [change] process. However, if the interests of various actors coincide, the outcome will be more successful if the powerful group uses consultation and seeks the views of others who are affected.
2. When power is concentrated in a small group but interests conflict, there may be no feasible strategy but [to attempt] unilateral command.
3. When power is diffused among many actors and their interests coincide, a strategy of joint participation will be effective in generating a solution supported by everyone.
4. When power is diffused among many actors but their interests conflict, a strategy of bargaining will be required. Compromise is inevitable and the outcome uncertain.

In most EMS systems joint participation is the best implementation strategy. The importance of the actors cannot be underestimated in the change process. This is why the new quality programs that encourage worker-management cooperation have been so successful.

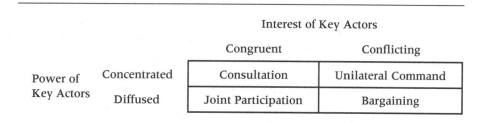

Power of Key Actors		Interest of Key Actors	
		Congruent	Conflicting
Power of Key Actors	Concentrated	Consultation	Unilateral Command
	Diffused	Joint Participation	Bargaining

Figure 5-1 Implementation strategies. (Adapted from Munson FC, Pelz DC: Innovating in organizations: a conceptual framework, unpublished manuscript, 1982.)

Key Features of an Innovation

As described in the preceding section the excellence of an innovation does not ensure the success of the change process. Besides the core content the salient features of an innovation are its originality, its political impact, and its technical complexity. Munson and Pelz[6] propose the following about the originality of an innovation:

1. The more original the solution, the longer the [change] process is likely to be and the more unforeseen difficulties will be encountered.
2. The more original the solution, the more time and attention must be paid to [the] stages of diagnosis and design. If implementation is attempted too quickly, the risk of failure is high.
3. The more original the solution, the more a small-scale pilot test will be needed to allow for rediagnosis and redesign. If large scale or systemwide implementation is hurriedly attempted, the risk of failure is high.

These proposals support one's intuition and have empirically been tested many times. For example, it is often easier to adapt a borrowed protocol from a similar EMS system than to start from the beginning.

Even the best innovation can fail if its political impact is not understood. The following principles are noteworthy:

1. Any behavior or technique that has come to symbolize a worker's identity will be difficult to change [i.e., high-speed driving with lights and sirens].
2. Similarly, learning a new innovation is more difficult if the behavior or technique it replaces is highly valued.
3. An innovation that has no effect or has a positive effect on one's self-image will be easier to implement.[5]

Encouraging the affected providers to contribute to the content of an innovation in the design stage reduces opposition and any negative political impact.

Although politics are often the most significant obstacle to the change process, the technical content of an innovation may also present problems. Difficulties in learning a complex procedure, such as prehospital 12-lead EKGs, can be overcome by investments in training methods and materials. As the preparation for an innovation increases, the difficulties in implementing it should decrease.[5] Also, proper preparation and packaging of an innovation lessen its political impact on the change process. Close attention must be paid to the key features of any innovation: originality, political impact, and complexity. These features can be manipulated to help persuade the powerful actors. However, all innovations need not be loved; some need only be tolerated.[5]

Key Features of an Organization

The organization must be prepared to change. An atmosphere must exist in which the participants are allowed to take the required actions throughout the change process.[5] Organizational policies must afford employees the latitude to participate in the diagnosis, design, and implementation of an innovation. This is the focus of the new quality programs. Munson and Pelz[5] also provide guidelines in this area:

1. When those who implement an innovation have also designed it, organizational preparation has already begun in the design stage.
2. To prepare the organization, it is necessary to present the content and purpose of the innovation to those with power and potential interest.

An innovation should not be perceived as a surprise to anyone within the organization. A steering committee comprised of powerful actors can be beneficial in communicating and preparing the organization for change. In an EMS system this may include not only the medical director and the providers but also the hospital administrators and the community representatives.

Role of a Pilot Introduction

In final preparation for the change process a pilot introduction of an innovation may be useful. Pilot introductions also give the organization the opportunity to concentrate its resources on an innovation's success.

> A small-scale introduction strongly suggests an approach that is experimental, tentative, developmental. Changes in the innovation are expected and are evidence of openness and flexibility, rather than of planning mistakes and sloppy design. For a similar reason it is desirable to choose a location where the likelihood of success is high. It is important to the final success of the implementation that the organization can see, and the implementors can experience, a successful operation.[5]

The evaluation of the pilot introduction is best done by a group process. Often, such groups arise spontaneously if not formed by the organization.[5] These gripe sessions, authorized or not, can have a profound effect on the outcome of the trial and the future implementation of the innovation. It is recommended that a formal review committee be established to help members deal with the stresses caused by using the unfamiliar innovation and to identify needed modifications.[5] Evaluation methods and criteria should be considered and discussed during the design stage and formalized prior to the initiation of the pilot. Expect rediagnosis and redesign to occur, keeping in mind that change is a process, not an event.

When the pilot introduction is successful, definitive systemwide implementation of an innovation can begin. Depending on the innovation, this may be a slow process. Continued communication with the review committee is required to ensure survivability and incorporation of the innovation—the definition of a successful innovation.

Summary

The arduous change process in EMS has begun. Current QA programs and research investigations are inadequate. Innovations are needed to unfreeze the current systems. The success of the change process depends on the implementation and survivability of these innovations. Although each innovation has unique qualities, fundamental characteristics exist that can be manipulated to assist in its successful implementation. The application of conditional principles that are based on understanding the key actors' power and interest should be used to direct the implementation strategy. Successful implementation cannot occur, however, until an EMS system realizes that change is necessary to deliver excellent prehospital care. It is hoped that the new quality programs will foster this view, and the change process will begin with the successful implementation of an innovation.

ACKNOWLEDGMENT

The author thanks Professor Fred Munson for reviewing this chapter.

REFERENCES

1. Berwick DM: *Curing health care: New strategies for quality improvement,* San Francisco, 1990, Jossey-Bass.
2. Deming WE: *Out of the crisis,* Cambridge, Mass, 1986 Massachusetts Institute of Technology—Center for Advanced Engineering Study.
3. Lewin K: Frontiers in group dynamics, *Human Relations* 1:5-41, 1947.
4. Morgan G: *Images of Organization,* London, 1986, Sage.
5. Munson FC, Pelz DC: Innovating in organizations: a conceptual framework, unpublished manuscript, 1982.
6. Pelz DC, Munson FC: A framework for organizational innovating. Proceedings of the international conference of Participatory Approaches to Improving Workplace Health, Labor Studies Center, University of Michigan, Ann Arbor, Mich, June 3-5, 1991.
7. Senge PM: The leaders new work: building learning organizations, *Sloan Management Review* 32:7-23, 1990.

6

Closing the Loop: Discard Bad Apples or Continuously Improve EMS?

Steven J. Davidson, M.D.

Directing change is the essence of management. Using the information gained in studying a system to change behavior within that system results in "closing the loop."

There are many means of effecting change, once the need for change is recognized and the type of change is determined. Methods, both authoritarian and participative, are widely practiced in enterprises worldwide, including medical practice and emergency medical services (EMS) systems. The initial structure of the quality improvement (QI) program, the continuing commitment of top management, and the participation of all system members are crucial to the ability of the program to effect change.

This chapter discusses two paradigms of management, or closing the loop. A rather traditional, authoritarian approach of closing the loop through a "cycle of fear" is contrasted with a less widely known but highly successful participatory model that is frequently credited with the success of modern-day Japanese industry. This latter model is gaining broad interest throughout health care. The "Deming Cycle," as it is widely known, offers many potential benefits to EMS system managers; an explanation of these advantages and a process for introducing continuous improvement conclude this chapter.

Traditional Approach: Inspect and Repair, or Discard

The preceding chapters have described a variety of approaches for gathering data, thereby allowing for evaluation of various aspects of the EMS system. System managers in quality assurance (QA) programs are conducting inspections of system structure, process, and outcome in a hunt for outliers, cases and individuals that lie outside of some explicit or implicit limit. The methodologies described in earlier chapters are directed toward identification of outliers. In EMS we are particularly prone to identify single occurrences through case reviews, an anecdotal method that attempts to flag instances of deviation from patient-care protocols or policies. Through this process we identify individuals who we believe need "fixing," although we often use euphemisms, such as "education" or "attitude adjustment."

The underlying theory behind this type of QA activity presupposes a "hunt for bad apples." We cloak our efforts in scientific methods and reporting since we characterize our endeavor as a search for those who fall more than some multiple of the standard deviation below the mean of some measure of quality (Figure 6-1).

Once we've identified the outliers, we then move to close the loop by somehow modifying their behavior. Subsequently, we measure the population again and identify a new batch of outliers. Because of the inevitable range of human performance, there will always be some outliers, since our theory includes the use of some cutoff point. Human nature and capacities being what they are, it is inevitable that sooner or later we will find one or more individuals who are consistently not measuring up to the specification.

IDENTIFICATION OF OUTLIERS

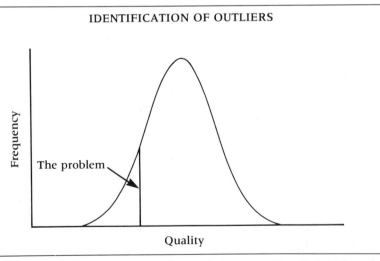

Figure 6-1 EMS providers who provide low-quality care are identified. (Adapted from National Demonstration Project Syllabus on Quality Improvement in Health Care, Brookline, Mass.)

Traditional Approach: Current Methods and Examples

Categories of QA actions in closing the loop include the following:
- actions on the system
- actions on personnel within the system
- continued observation of the system and system personnel

Positive feedback actions on the system and system personnel are intended to be reinforcing to encourage continued excellence. Other actions on the system and system personnel, neither explicitly negative nor positive, may attempt to alter behavior through rational processes, i.e., through further training of system personnel or alteration of long-standing system policies that no longer serve a need. Lastly, negative actions on the system and system personnel may be punitive, i.e., disciplinary in nature for personnel or organizational components.

Effective Communications

Communication in a reliable and consistent manner is necessary to convey to personnel the feedback message, whether the message is specific to an individual or broadly focused on system issues.[8] System managers too often assume that the authority of their position entitles them to communicate to workers using methods that are most efficient for them. Unfortunately, the means of communication of feedback and the manner of that communication can either accentuate or dilute the message itself. The most effective system managers seek the assistance of system personnel to determine the strengths and effectiveness of their communications.[9] System managers can thus gain some assurance that the feedback offered will not lose effectiveness because of the manner of its delivery.

What kind of feedback is appropriate and when? Currently, most medical directors use an informal method of positive feedback by praising individual providers, usually one on one. Annual fund-raising or recognition events may single out a small number of providers or units. Systematic reward and recognition is the exception.

Negative feedback tends to be more systematized because of the necessity of due process should negative findings lead to discipline, demotion, or discharge. Undesirable processes and results often lead to further training, which is then misconstrued by system personnel as a form of negative feedback. Administrative system managers frequently convey this message to field providers since the costs of additional training are an expense to the ambulance service. Beyond additional training interventions, disciplinary interventions of several sorts are commonly employed.

Unionized, civil-service municipal agencies are generally the most structured in their approach to intervention and feedback. Positive feedback is generally freely bestowed, but negative feedback is afforded through only the most structured of processes. An example of this process follows.

The Philadelphia Fire Department's (PFD) Division of EMS accepts complaints from the community at large, the fire department's members and officers, the medical community, and the quality process supervised by the system medical director. All are pursued in the same consistent fashion. Issues that do not involve patients or medical policies and practices in any way (i.e., those originating in the fire house) are managed without the involvement of the medical director; all other incidents are shared with the system medical director.

Information about the incident is collected using all available records: trip sheets, medical command records, tape-recorded online medical command, hospital reports, etc. Field providers may then be queried in person or over the telephone by paramedic training and evaluation staff who report to the system medical director. Depending on whether or not the patient or patients involved were at risk of injury as a result of the paramedic's action, the inquiry may proceed at either "level I" or "level II." Level I inquiries are frequently conducted for protocol deviations, most commonly for errors of commission, such as occasions in which the paramedic(s) exceeded usual drug-dosage guidelines without benefit of an online physician order. Failure to obtain medical command on a patient nontransport is another example.

More serious incidents, including drug-administration incidents involving controlled drugs and errors of omission, are managed at level II, which entails an in-person meeting with both paramedic training and evaluation staff and a PFD EMS officer. Paramedics involved in a level II investigation are advised they may have union representation at the meeting, since they may have participated in a case with a bad patient outcome believed to have occurred as a result of their own malfeasance. Independent reports are developed by the PFD EMS officer and the medical director's staff representative and reviewed by the director of EMS, a PFD deputy chief, and the medical director. They consult, and either the director or the medical director may recommend proceeding to level III, where together they personally interview the paramedics involved in the presence of union representation. This meeting can result in an oral and/or written reprimand. Further disciplinary action results only if charges are filed and the standard PFD disciplinary process is pursued.

Level I and level II inquiries generally result in educational and monitoring interventions. Escalation of usual level I inquiries to level II for repeat offenders has been used with some apparent effectiveness since the presence of the PFD officer adds considerable weight to the advice and the training intervention offered by the medical director's staff member.

The filing of formal charges results in the convening of a hearing panel that can recommend discipline, including suspension without pay for varying intervals, demotion, or discharge. The deputy chief has expressed his willingness to file charges in appropriate cases. As of the date of this writing, one case has gone to a hearing panel resulting in suspensions for the providers involved. As an alternative route, the medical director has the authority under state law and regulation to suspend a paramedic's authorization to care for patients; at the present time, this action has been used sparingly and only in concert with the process previously described.

The Problem We All Face

This disciplinary focus of a QA program is fraught with problems. Each of us knows that every system harbors a "worst medic." What should one do at this point? Should we fire our worst medic, thereby adhering to our standard? Will this motivate the remainder of the work force to work harder and perform better, or will we be left with some other individual to now fill the position of "bad apple," and will we have to go through the process all over again with him or her?

What usually happens in such instances is that the status quo is effectively reinforced and a defensive reaction develops on the part of the work force. They all respond, "My apple is just fine, thank you. Go away and look at somebody else's apple." This predictable defensive reaction feeds into a cycle of fear (Figure 6-2).

Workers, field professionals, paraprofessionals, and support personnel alike view quality interventions that seek bad apples as a measure of increased observation on the part of system managers. In effect, they view these efforts as symptomatic of a basic mistrust of the work force by the system managers. The work force comes to fear management, viewing system managers as concerned only with evidence of aberrant behavior. Workers do not turn to system managers for support and direction since they begin to fear that their questions and concerns about system performance will be viewed as a weakness. They come to fear being the messenger of ill tidings.

Subsequently, all audits, inspections, and other quality activities come to be viewed with suspicion by workers, who perceive the underlying message as being directed toward themselves as individuals, not toward system improvement. Therefore they begin to manipulate the system, since individually they want system managers to perceive that everything is just fine with them. We as system managers, too smart to be fooled by such efforts, consequently redouble our efforts to assure ourselves that we are not overlooking a serious problem, although we are actually creating one.

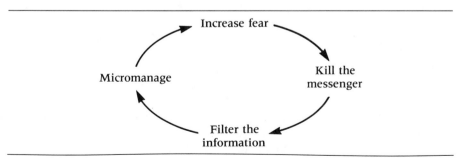

Figure 6-2 Evoked by a defensive reaction, the cycle of fear maintains the status quo. (Adapted from Scherkenbach WW: *The Deming route to quality and productivity,* Washington, DC, 1986, CEEPress Books, George Washington University.)

What you get at this point is a system that may appear to be holding itself together on paper, but worker dissatisfaction is a potent time bomb that can precipitate inadequate service as measured by patient and community satisfaction.

W. Edwards Deming and Management for Quality

W. Edwards Deming, a statistician who pioneered applying methods of statistical process control to manufacturing industry during the 1940s, was recognized by Japan in 1960 with the Second Order of the Sacred Treasure—the first American ever to receive such an honor. Over the last decade Dr. Deming has gained renown in his own country for proclaiming the necessity for a complete management overhaul in the United States. His ideas have begun to be embraced throughout industry, including the service sector. At age 90, he continues to present his program to new audiences.

Medicine has begun to recognize the potential of the Deming management method. The National Demonstration Project on Quality Improvement in Health Care (NDP on QI in Health Care), funded by grants from the John A. Hartford Foundation, has developed an investigative and training program operating out of the Harvard School of Public Health and the Institute for Healthcare Improvement.[2] Large health-care provider systems, including the Harvard Community Health Plan and the Henry Ford System, have adopted Deming's methodologies and are implementing quality activities consistent with the Deming management method.

An insistence on defining quality by the consumer or product user is intrinsic to the Deming management method as described in Chapter 1. In EMS, dimensions of quality might include patient outcome (e.g., survival from cardiac arrest), interpersonal relations, integration into the community's health-care system, patient access, and pride among workers. Jack Stout has championed the need for consistency and reliability of performance for an EMS system to be considered "high performance."[10] Other dimensions of quality may be substituted or added as long as measures are aimed at evaluating an aspect of quality relevant to EMS system customers, primarily our patients. Deming and others also describe "internal customers" who are dependent on the work of other members of the system. For example, field providers are dependent on the performance of dispatchers, who themselves may depend on the work of the complaint-taker who actually speaks to the citizen requesting assistance.

If the true mission of an EMS system is to provide quality care to patients, then the theory of continuous improvement may serve as a tool system managers employ to achieve reliable quality. However, this presupposes that Deming's transformation applies equally to EMS, that we do in fact have reliable quality as our constant purpose and are not interested in quality merely as something tacked on, an outrigger required by an outside agency.

Deming's call for a management transformation includes specific features that require attention: both those needing a positive emphasis, i.e., *The Fourteen*

Points, and those requiring a negative emphasis, i.e., *The Seven Deadly Diseases.* These constitute the principles on which Deming's transformation of management is predicated, as described in Chapter 2. These principles, embodied in the theory of continuous improvement, can be applied not only to the mechanical operations of ambulance maintenance but also to the medical care provided by an EMS system. Berwick,[1] a leading spokesperson for continuous quality improvement (CQI) in health care, has supported the application of continuous improvement to EMS. The application of this paradigm to health care has been described in detail.[2]

Although it is impossible to encapsulate the entire content of Dr. Deming's thesis in a single chapter, it should become clear that confusion by a system manager can confound his or her best efforts to effectively close the loop and effect positive change. These best efforts may in fact make things worse.

Continuous Improvement: Every Defect is a Treasure

If, instead of hunting for bad apples, all EMS workers are impressed with the idea that every defect is a treasure that provides an opportunity to learn more about the EMS system, then workers become empowered and able to participate in system learning. Rather than being objects on whom system managers employ quality activities, workers become collaborators in efforts at QI.

Each problem provides an occasion to determine if the EMS system is under control or out of control. In EMS, each defect or problem may have a deleterious impact on one or more patients. No theory of management can minimize the impact to the patient and community thus injured. However, system managers have a responsibility, beyond the individual patient, to ensure that the EMS system extracts the maximum amount of knowledge from the experience. Every process in every system provides information that can be used to examine the process to determine if it is meeting its real goal.

Through learning about a process, EMS system managers can distinguish between a stable and an unstable system. A stable system is, by definition, a system under control, regardless of how variably it performs. To reach stability the system must discover and remove the special causes of trouble, the defects. Many methods—including control charts, Pareto charts, Ishikawa charts ("cause and effect" or "fishbone diagram") and others (see Deming,[4] Brassard,[3] and Small[12])—can be applied through the Shewhart-Deming cycle to help reveal these special causes of trouble (Figure 6-3).

Ultimately, when the causes of trouble have been removed and the system is performing in a stable fashion, the same methods can assist in improving overall system performance by assisting system managers in examining the causes of intrinsic system variability. Ultimately, these efforts will result in continuous improvement and system evolution (Figure 6-4).

One may then draw the corollary that a stable system with a high degree of variability is not the responsibility of workers since system variability and its reduction are responsibilities of system managers. Hunting for bad apples in a

SHEWHART-DEMING CYCLE

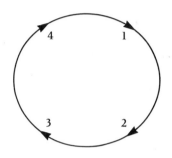

1. What could be the most important accomplishments of this effort? What changes might be desirable? What data are available? Are new observations needed? If yes, plan a change or test. Decide how to use the observations.

2. Carry out the change or test decided upon, preferably on a small scale.

3. Observe the effects of the change or test.

4. Study the results. What did we learn? What can we predict?

5. Repeat step 1, with knowledge accumulated.

6. Repeat step 2, and onward.

Figure 6-3 Analytical tools applied through the Shewart-Deming cycle result in CQI. (Adapted from Deming WE: *Out of the crisis,* Cambridge, 1986, MIT Center for Advanced English Study.)

stable system with high variability does identify outliers (those at the extremes of a highly variable but stable system), but it is the system, *not* the willing worker who is doing his best, that is responsible for the particular outcome. The system itself produces a real and measurable number of defects.

Dr. Deming points to two mistakes that result in loss when system managers confuse special causes of problems with common causes of problems:

Mistake 1: Ascribe a variation or a mistake to a special cause (e.g., the medic-nurse relationship) when in fact the cause belongs to system variability (e.g., the common cause of the time interval to restock the unit).

Mistake 2: Ascribe a variation or a mistake to system variability (i.e., common causes) when in fact the cause was special. (The reverse of mistake number 1.)

The data collected to serve traditional quality processes may not support the CQI process and may in fact increase problems. Counting defects in and of itself is useless unless the range of behavior for the specific process under study is known. Therefore system managers who pursue every incident as if it results from a special—or unique—defect may be mistaking high system variability for special causes of a particular problem. Unless system managers determine the control limits of processes in their system, however, how could they know the difference? (See Chapter 11.)

CONTINUOUS IMPROVEMENT

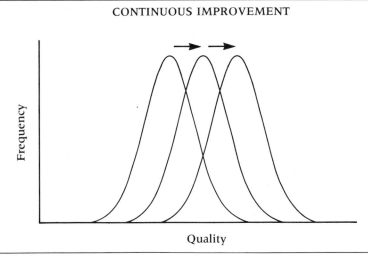

Figure 6-4 When problem identification impels continuous improvement, outliers aren't dropped, rather everything (and everybody) gets better. (Adapted from National Demonstration Project Syllabus on Quality Improvement in Health Care, Brookline, Mass.)

Constant adjustment, such as intervening with a paramedic in every case of apparent deviation from protocol, is an example of mistake number one. Ignoring a problem, such as overlooking the failure of a piece of equipment because "it happens rarely," is an example of mistake two.

High system variability often results from an unclear purpose. The EMS system that purports to have as its purpose immediate quality prehospital care of the acutely ill or injured may, for example, convey to workers the message that the system purpose is to maintain the average response time under 6 minutes. Thus workers may race to calls of low urgency to maintain an overall low average-response time, resulting in dangerous driving and excessive vehicle wear and tear. Effective leadership requires a clearly articulated constancy of purpose directed to the true organizational mission.

Occasionally, poor job design contributes to poor system performance. For example, field supervisors may be so overburdened with administrative responsibility that they themselves are unable to respond to cardiac-arrest cases or multiple casualties and thus are unable to serve as role models and leaders for less experienced field providers. The ongoing shortage of paramedics in much of the country may lead a system manager to push trainees through an intensive training program in too brief a time span. The inadequate training that results may be manifested by inconsistent or even absent field performance of psychomotor skills and inaccurate field assessments.

System managers are responsible for any lack of clarity regarding the system's mission and for educational or job orientation programs that are irrelevant to the real job; they are responsible for improving the system. If the medical director lacks the authority to direct the change, he can serve as a teacher and, through the physician-educator role, educate administrative partners to recognize the necessity for the transformation. Through education and the use of successful small-scale examples, change can be introduced most successfully. The converse may also apply should the system administrator be motivated to improve the system and a complacent medical director is inhibiting change.

Listening to field workers and system support workers can be the key to uncovering any defects. Their experience in rendering the hands-on service—whether to patients or to ambulances—can assist system managers in identifying the cause of the trouble. For example, field providers may report that patient extrications from motor vehicles are taking too long because the proper equipment is damaged or missing or because inexperienced extrication personnel have been substituted for experienced staff members. By identifying the specific problem, they direct attention to parameters that management should measure, facilitating identification of the root causes of system variability.

The experience of participating in this fashion empowers workers by underlining their ability to improve the system. Workers bring their observations and experience to the fore; this helps management decide what to study through the Shewhart-Deming cycle, and often the attempted improvement or "fix" originates from workers' suggestions. The use and application of the cycle, a management responsibility, provides workers with a method that helps them improve system performance. Together, worker and manager go forward continuously improving EMS.

Continuous Improvement Applied

Many systems set specific requirements for turnaround time, i.e., time out of service at the hospital following patient delivery. Enlightened systems may permit more than one "standard" time. For example, a routine case may be permitted 30 minutes for cleaning up, restocking, and recordkeeping; following a code or trauma case the crew may be permitted up to an hour to accomplish these tasks. If tracked, this period is often compared to the permitted time, a specification usually determined in arbitrary fashion or by best estimate of a reasonable interval.

In a system of continuous improvement, this interval would be measured and control limits computed. Different control charts could be constructed for each receiving hospital or category of patient or medic team. In any case, the upper and lower control limits would be computed and used as a basis for determining future interventions. Once the interval is determined to be stable and within the control limits, sampling at intervals, perhaps no more than once a month (depending on the frequency of service) would then be adequate to determine if the system is stable. If the turnaround time on any case exceeded the upper control limit, then the special cause should be sought immediately (Figure 6-5).

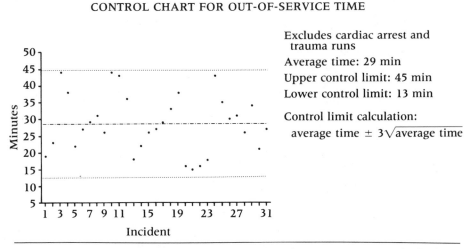

CONTROL CHART FOR OUT-OF-SERVICE TIME

Excludes cardiac arrest and trauma runs
Average time: 29 min
Upper control limit: 45 min
Lower control limit: 13 min

Control limit calculation:
$$\text{average time} \pm 3\sqrt{\text{average time}}$$

Figure 6-5 Each incident is plotted against the out-of-service time to reveal whether this provider at this specific hospital is within system limits.

For example, if ambulance turnaround time at a specific receiving hospital is noted to be overlong at certain times, a control chart that plots duration of time at the hospital against date and time might reveal a pattern. That pattern might indicate that the unit had a prolonged (outside of control limits) time whenever a certain medic took a patient to the hospital when a certain nurse was working. The relationship between the medic and the nurse denotes a special cause of trouble: an overlong time at the hospital.

Because a turnaround time with high variability may adversely affect system performance by resulting in queued calls and delayed ambulance response to an emergency, system managers may wish to reduce the average turnaround time and the variability. Once the system is seen to be stable as in the example cited, no amount of exhortation to the paramedics will result in a decreased time; in fact, tampering in this fashion may worsen results. Instead, careful examination of what occurs when Medic Unit *Q* arrives at Mount Elsewhere Hospital can identify aspects of the system that can be improved to reduce the average turnaround time.

For example, if the average time at the hospital following transport of a seriously injured trauma patient is consistently and reliably 1 hour and always falls within the control limits, the system is stable and reliable. However, the 1-hour turnaround time might stress the system by requiring adjacent units to respond into the out-of-service unit's primary response zone. System managers may find this unacceptable and prefer a shorter interval spent at the hospital. Using a cause-and-effect diagram, the methods, the manpower, the material, and the machinery that compose the work effort at the hospital during the turnaround time might be clarified. Through field provider input, it may become apparent that restocking of the ambulance after a trauma run is extensive and time-consuming. The use of a prepackaged trauma restocking kit might save substantial time and at the same time improve the hospital's inventorying and billing for the restocking. In addition, the EMS system would gain a consistently and reliably shorter turnaround time for trauma runs at that hospital, thereby improving availability of the unit in its primary response zone.

Similar methods may be applied to the many other activities in which duration of activities may be relevant. However, the reader is cautioned not to oversimplify complex circumstances. For example, duration of scene management of a cardiac-arrest patient is probably not a useful effort. The variability is bound to be large, unless the data are divided into many small cells representing apparent contributors to duration of time on scene. Of course the number of available data points then may become too small to be of value.

When an EMS system manager closes the loop in this fashion, he puts aside preconceived notions and specifications and begins thinking in terms of a total system that includes components outside of the EMS manager's control, such as the emergency department staff, supplies, and telephone availability. This kind of "system thinking" requires a broad view and interaction with the entire range of system components. Dr. Deming[5] refers to this as "profound knowledge," a "putting together components of a system for optimization of the system."

Continuous Improvement in EMS: Why?

Our responsibility to our patients causes us to seek means by which we can continuously improve and provide quality medical care that is perceived as such by both patients and providers. Continuous improvement applied to health care in general and EMS in particular focuses on patients and thus coincides with the primary motivator for those of us in the helping professions.

EMS professionals and paraprofessionals need not be exhorted to improve their work. By and large, those who enter the helping professions such as EMS do so because the responsibility for service to sick and injured people corresponds with their individual ethos. Surely we all work for money, but the rewards of our profession exceed the mere pecuniary.

Yet increasingly, health-care managers, including those in EMS, focus on our workers as a means of responding to society's increased demand for accountability in the provision of health care. Traditional QA activities that emphasize individual workers have heightened sensitivities and brought defensive reactions to interactions that previously had been occasions for mutual learning. Hospital-based, EMS-focused morbidity and mortality conferences are conducted in formats approved by hospital lawyers so as not to pose a legal risk to providers. Together the result has been a demeaning of physicians, nurses, and field providers alike. Finger pointing is now commonplace where once collegial relations were the rule. Broadening our mutual perspective through the concept of profound knowledge and applying the theory of CQI enable management and workers to refocus their efforts together on the real work of improving patient care and outcome. This also reduces the narrow focus on individual workers, which leads to the detriment of all.

As all work together to improve the system—and it does improve—all reap benefits. Pride among system workers is echoed in the community, which recognizes the improvements in the EMS system. The system becomes better able to argue for and obtain increased economic support. Lastly, current and likely future economic realities for public service being what they are, a CQI program holds out the hope of improving operational efficiencies so that even if costs cannot be reduced in bulk, the rate of growth in operating costs can be reduced.

Continuous Improvement in EMS: How Can We Get It?

Senior EMS system managers must commit to continuous improvement if more than temporary gains are to be achieved. Outside sources must be sought to help system managers achieve the profound knowledge, the broad-system viewpoint, that will be critical to the new way of operating required by CQI. This new management culture will necessitate that system managers become severely and acutely uncomfortable with the status quo. They will have to grope toward the new way, and those who are comfortable with things as they stand will be unwilling to expend the effort. Often, a junior manager can help a senior manager recognize how seriously disordered their present EMS system has become. By bringing forth a small example that the junior manager has accomplished, the necessary senior leadership can be developed. But senior-level commitment, which includes personal responsibility and accountability on the part of the senior manager, is critical to the transformation.

This new management culture requires that system managers develop perspectives that are particularly difficult, especially for health-care workers. Inherent variability in the EMS system will inevitably result in less salutary outcomes for some patients. In the long run, efforts will be bent toward reducing system variability. Initially, though, as system managers determine control limits of various processes, they will have to accept these "bad" outcomes and be especially diligent not to give in to tampering. Efforts to recognize and correct special causes of problems must continue, indeed be redoubled. However, occurrences of bad outcome that fall within control limits of processes under evaluation must not be an excuse for return to traditional patterns of searching for an outlier; rather, they must provide the motivation for continuing to eliminate special causes of variability so that the common causes of variability (i.e., those inherent in the present system) can ultimately be effectively addressed.

Profound knowledge and new skills for examining and understanding processes can be gleaned from many sources. Among the best for those of us in EMS are our colleagues in other service industries who have made the commitment to CQI. Often, local chambers of commerce have groups devoted to QI, and these groups can be a source of general information. The references cited at the end of this chapter, continuing education courses offered through professional associations, and course work on CQI in local business schools can also be useful resources.

Ultimately the knowledge and skills gained must be applied to each system individually. Each time marks a new experiment since no two systems respond alike. In general, one must develop a strategy for transforming the EMS system to a system of CQI. It is not possible that all will change overnight; Dr. Deming speaks of 5 years or more as the required commitment. Furthermore, the larger the initial impact sought, the riskier is the effort. Starting with a small component that can be encompassed within the grasp of a single senior manager who is committed to the effort is a more sensible strategy. A successful demonstration project, no matter how small, begins the necessary process of persuading doubters that system management is committed to the change and that the transformation is possible. The longest journey begins with but a single step.

The changes in EMS systems necessitated by the introduction of CQI are fundamental and threatening. In all environments multiple interests collide, and conflict gives rise to politics. Whenever possible, prevent confrontation, not by ignoring or avoiding important issues but rather by converting win-lose conflict into win-win partnerships. For example, fire chiefs and medical directors usually share the same goal: good patient care. However, the constituencies that judge, interpret, and publicize the attainment of this goal differ and often use varying measuring sticks. Therefore allowing the fire chief, the mayor, the city council, and the political process to evaluate that which they can while the medical community evaluates data within its area of expertise tends to bring the fire chief and the medical director together rather than driving them apart. Naturally, starting with such a global goal is nearly impossible, and this approach is best taken with a small start.

The politics of EMS, with its profusion of interested parties, results in change measured on a "glacial time scale."[6] Patience and persistent patient advocacy ultimately produce the desired result.[11] It is important to remember that being political is part of the EMS medical director's role when exerted toward patient advocacy. Playing politics to maintain a constituency among elected officials, bureaucrats, and influential citizens is counterproductive.

Summary

Managers have a panoply of techniques they can employ to induce change in an EMS system. They may choose to select an authoritarian system, dependent on inspection and continuous supervision with a resulting tendency toward micromanagement. This approach, focusing as it does on individuals and their efforts, gives rise to exhortation of the workforce on the one hand and to discipline of the individuals on the other. The search for outliers this approach entails gives rise to a myriad of unintended actions, all of which result in increased activities at the expense of accomplishing real work.

In medicine we've begun to incorporate the patient's assessment of quality through outcomes management.[7] Patient-management protocols for field providers hold the promise of serving as descriptors of the process of prehospital patient care. Statistical process-control techniques—described by Shewhart, refined by Deming, brought to medicine through the NDP on QI in Health Care, and adopted by all of us in transforming our EMS systems—hold the promise of assuring high-quality patient care.

The Deming system, which seeks to direct attention to the system of work and not to the individual worker or work force as a whole, provides the opportunity to understand sources and the extent of system variability. This results in system refinements and higher productivity (quality and effectiveness) since workers work smarter, not harder. Workers, aware of the process, have the opportunity to have more and greater pride in their work, thus tending through peer pressure to become the kind of work force system managers sought in the first place: a work force full of pride because of consistent performance, which is directed at continuous improvement of dimensions of quality medical care.

In the 1990s the communities we serve and the professionals within our EMS systems demand high-quality prehospital care. This transformation can only be accomplished by abandoning supervision and the hunt for bad apples. It is time to embrace leadership and continuous improvement of EMS.

REFERENCES

1. Berwick DM: Sounding board: continuous improvement as an ideal in health care, *N Engl J Med* 320:53-56, 1989.
2. Berwick DM, Godfrey AB, Roessner J: *Curing health care: new strategies for quality improvement,* San Francisco, 1990, Jossey-Bass.
3. Brassard M: *The memory jogger plus +*™, Methuen, 1989, GOAL/QPC.
4. Deming WE: *Out of the crisis,* Cambridge, 1986, MIT Center for Advanced Engineering Study.
5. Deming WE: *Transformation for management of quality and productivity.* The Philadelphia Area Council for Excellence, Philadelphia, February 19-22, 1991.
6. Dinerman N:˷ *Putting it together—Political choreography,* EMS Medical Director's Course, NAEMSP, Orlando, Fla, June 1991.
7. Elwood PM: Shattuck lecture—Outcomes management: a technology of patient experience, *N Engl J Med* 318:1549-1556, 1988.
8. Ende J: Feedback in clinical medical education, *JAMA* 250:777-781, 1983.
9. Miller JR, Lewis FM: Closing the gap in quality assurance: a tool for evaluating group leaders, *Health Educ Q* 9:55-66, 1982.
10. National EMS Medical Director's Course, National Association of EMS Physicians sixth annual meeting, Houston, June 13-14, 1990.
11. Pepe PE: *Administration of emergency medical services.* In Manning JE, Williams JM, editors: *Resident guide to pursuing an academic career in emergency medicine,* Dallas, 1992, Society of Academic Emergency Medicine and the Emergency Medicine Residents' Association.
12. Small BB: *Statistical quality control handbook,* ed 2, Indianapolis, 1985, AT&T Technologies.

7

Implementing Quality Management

Andrew G. Wilson, Jr., M.D.

The principles of continuous quality improvement (CQI) have been discussed in the preceding chapters of this book. The application of these principles to lead an organization may be referred to as quality management (QM). Simply put, QM is the "decriminalization" of quality issues. With a 40-year history of successful application in industry, QM has recently been applied to health care.

Although not been widely applied to the prehospital arena, emergency medical services (EMS) should be fertile ground for QM. Most EMS systems are interorganizational, involving at least two and often many different organizations (e.g., police, fire, private provider, and hospital). Although the search for "bad apples" and attendant finger-pointing engendered by QA is poorly tolerated within a single organization, it is exponentially more difficult to accommodate among different organizations. Although there is a strong commonality of purpose (i.e., high-quality patient care) among the different organizations comprising an EMS system, it is often difficult to discuss obstacles to quality care without inspiring defensiveness and hostility. QM offers a means of peaceably breaching the walls that may exist among EMS system components. This provides a tremendous theoretic advantage for the implementation of QM in EMS, and there are no theoretic barriers to its application.

The striking feature of QM's application to health care is just how relevant it really is. This chapter discusses EMS QM based on established industrial principles and emerging principles gleaned from health-care application.

Organizational Culture

Although it is easy to speak of implementing QM, just what is it that is being implemented? The answer is nothing short of a profound change in organizational culture. The culture of an organization is the sum total of the ways the affairs of that organization are conducted. The ways in which members of the organization view themselves and their customers, the manner in which management interacts with workers, and the ways in which workers interact with each other are all facets of an organization's culture. An organization may be described as being liberal or conservative, risk taking or cautious, paternalistic or autocratic, arrogant or contrite.

Whatever the culture of the organization at the outset of the QM implementation, all activities begin to be focused toward improving quality after implementation begins. Implementation of QM may mean different changes in different organizations, but all share elements in common. There is empowerment of workers to identify problems in processes and to make changes in those processes. There is recognition that customers, both internal and external to the organization, are always right. There is the acceptance of problems as opportunities to improve and not as opportunities to assign blame.

The benefits of producing the necessary changes should not be perceived as simply enhancing the quality of the product, but as also enhancing efficiency and cost savings for the organization. QM implementation must be viewed as a long-term commitment. It is not a gadget to be tried briefly and with scant commitment. Given the profound changes in an organization required for QM implementation, a concept of the framework of QM is helpful, as is the definition of some terms.

Total quality management (TQM) reflects the philosophy of management that enables quality improvement techniques throughout the organization. Because profound changes in an organization's culture are usually from the top down, the top leaders must subscribe to the philosophy of TQM and become educated in its principles.

Quality improvement (QI), although it may be construed more broadly, is the exercise of the principles of QM by teams constituted to address a given problem. QI teams, therefore, are the vehicle by which the actual work of QI is performed and from which changes in the processes of an organization occur.

Continuous Quality Improvement (CQI) is the action corollary of the TQM philosophy. An important tenet of TQM is that quality is amenable to continuous improvement. That is, the tools of QI are to be applied continuously to processes and problems within an organization.

Quality Management (QM) is used as a generic term in this chapter to connote aspects of TQM, CQI, and QI.

The essential elements necessary to begin implementing TQM are a belief in the principles of QM by top leadership and the successful constitution and execution of teams on the worker or staff level.

Team Approach to Problem Solving

QI teams are a central element of QM, and in fact do the work and precipitate organizational changes. Because they are so pivotal in the execution of TQM, a brief description by analogy of how a team functions is useful. See Figure 7-1 below for a comparison of the function of a QI team with the process of patient care.

Several points need to be made about the analogy between the process of patient care and the QI team's "care" of a problem:

1. Both are driven by data. Just as we use data to drive our care of a patient, so must a team use data to drive its examination of a problem and to formulate recommendations for a solution.

2. The patient-care sequence illustrated is imprinted into the physician's thought process through many years of training. To follow the steps in sequence requires discipline; to omit a step is to jeopardize the care of the patient. So it is with a team. Although the temptation with a problem is to jump from knowledge of the problem and observable symptoms to recommended solutions, discipline must be maintained to proceed through all the steps in sequence to avoid inappropriate or incorrect problem solutions.

3. Note the use of reexamination in a QI team's functioning and the analogous follow-up visit in patient care. It is not enough to think that a solution to a problem is at hand. It must be shown—using data—that the solution is the appropriate one and is working.

4. In a sense QI is the rigorous and the disciplined application of common sense to a sick process rather than to a sick patient. The uncanny resemblance of our activities in caring for patients to those activities of a team caring for a process is not coincidental. Industry co-opted the physician thinking process for application to its problems. Industry is perplexed that we in health care have not applied our own principles of problem solving to administrative problems and to collective, as well as individual, patient-care problems.

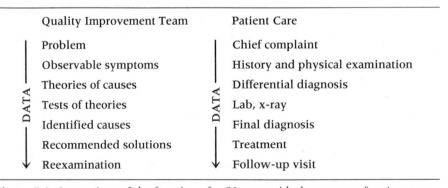

Quality Improvement Team	Patient Care
Problem	Chief complaint
Observable symptoms	History and physical examination
Theories of causes	Differential diagnosis
Tests of theories	Lab, x-ray
Identified causes	Final diagnosis
Recommended solutions	Treatment
Reexamination	Follow-up visit

Figure 7-1 Comparison of the function of a QI team with the process of patient care.

Implementing Quality Management

There are three general strategies for QM implementation within an organization: the organizationwide, top-down incremental, and bottom-up incremental approaches. Which strategy is chosen depends to a large degree on the attitudes and resources extant in a given organization. If the attitude of top management is enthusiastic, top management becomes involved at the outset, a distinct advantage. Resources, mostly financial, determine the rapidity of implementation. When the organization's leadership is enthusiastic, financial issues may slow but not preclude implementation.

In organizationwide training and implementation, top management is involved, committed, and educated. Then the remainder of the organization is educated and trained, as appropriate. During this process of education and training of the entire organization, no projects are initiated. Although in some respects this is the easiest approach, it is also the most expensive. It also poses the difficulty of sustaining enthusiasm throughout the organization as ideas are bandied about but no practical benefit is seen for the duration of the extended training period. Some hospitals, notably the Henry Ford Hospital System in Detroit and the University of Michigan, have undertaken this method of implementation.

The top-down incremental approach occupies a middle ground, and is the one most often chosen. In this model, top management is committed and becomes educated in the ways of QM. At this juncture, some focused pilot projects are undertaken. These pilot projects are carefully chosen for their high likelihood of success and visibility within the organization. The team members carrying out these pilot projects receive directed training. The training often can be "just in time" to provide the team members with the knowledge they need to go from step to step. On completion of successful pilot projects the top management and the organization capitalize on their successes, and the team projects grow in number, diversity, and degree of challenge. With continued successes, and inevitably some failures, the necessary cultural changes will occur within the organization as more and more people have experience with and subscribe to the principles of QM.

The bottom-up incremental approach may be tried when top management has not subscribed to the QM philosophy. As with any organizational endeavor lacking active top management support, QM in this setting is fraught with difficulties. For some organizations it may be the only way, and for some cultures it may be the best way. If this approach to implementation is attempted, the overall strategy is to field some successful teams and pique the interest of top management. Like the top-down incremental approach, this method builds on success. To be successful the managers involved should carefully choose projects on processes that are within their control to change.

Once the general strategy for QM implementation has been chosen, some general principles should be considered. However, the implementation process throughout related endeavors is much the same. The underlying principle of implementation may be summed as being the education of leadership and the institution of teams.

It is imperative when initiating implementation that leadership be thoroughly educated in the TQM philosophy and clear in their understanding of the principles of QM. Leadership must be committed to executing QI in the form of teams, with the necessary support and patience. They must adhere closely to the principles of QI team function. Extensive discussions of these principles are available in many references, but the reader may find Berwick's discussion[1] most relevant.

Leaders involved in the QM effort must cross all areas being examined by QI teams and must empower those individuals with the ability to change the organization and to implement the teams' recommendations. That is, if the leader of an important part of the organization is not willing to participate, QI efforts that involve that facet of the organization will likely fail. Leadership must reach to upper levels of management, and eventually to all levels of management, to effect acceptance of QM principles. Leadership must be willing to empower individuals at the staff or worker level if QI implementation is to succeed. This is one of the aspects of organizational-cultural change that proves most difficult for many individuals and organizations. If the leadership charges a team with examining a process and developing recommendations for improving it, the leadership must be willing to accede to the team's recommendations for change. This is not nearly as dangerous as might be thought, because the team function, when carried out correctly, involves responsible suggestions, and suggestions are backed by data that the leadership should find easy to accept.

The means by which the leadership of an EMS organization becomes educated is, simply put, to read and then to go. First, it is useful to have all the leaders expose themselves to the same general philosophy of TQM by reading many of the same materials. Again, Berwick[1] offers an excellent introduction that can serve as a QA outline for the leaders of a health-care oriented organization. Next, the leaders, or at least some of them, should go to meetings to hear these principles more fully articulated and to obtain collateral views of the same issues. There are many meetings, both within industry and health care, with QM as a central focus. Health-care oriented attendees may find it most useful to attend health-care oriented meetings, as the presentations are most directly applicable to health-care operations.

Project Selection

After the leadership is educated, the next step for most organizations is to establish project teams to demonstrate feasibility and utility and to generate further interest in QM. Organization leadership must first identify and prioritize problems to be solved. Any organization capable of elementary introspection can identify problems. The challenge is first to identify and then to describe clearly a problem that is amenable to solution by a QI team. As with much else in QM, this process is simple, but it is not easy. Identification of problems may come from a number of sources: internal and external customers, QA programs, sentinel events, or other sources.

Identification of a project that is amenable to QI methodology is more difficult. Projects should be clearly definable and have a short time cycle to facilitate measurement. Projects should involve a process not already experiencing a major transition. Because early projects are used to build enthusiasm within an organization, it should be one that is of interest to employees in the organization (see Case Study). It should also be a relatively simple one with definable starting and finish points. As with many problems, a clear, concise definition of a problem statement may be surprisingly difficult. Refer to Berwick[1] and Scholtes[5] for a more complete discussion of project selection.

Team Charge and Composition

The problem statement evolved by the QM leadership circumscribes the team membership and effectively constitutes a team charge. There are generally three components of a team:

1. *Team leader*—This person should have a good overall view of the problem to be solved. The leader should have leadership qualities but should not necessarily be the ranking member of the team or from management.
2. *Team members*—These should people should be the ones who "own" the process under discussion. Usually, team members are actual line workers, whether physicians or dispatchers, for they must have an intimate working knowledge of the process under consideration. Managers can function as team members, but line workers usually fare better.
3. *Team facilitator*—This person should be familiar with QI team functions. Knowledge of the problem process is not critical for the facilitator; in fact, facilitators may be borrowed from other industries. The job of the facilitator is to quietly and unassumingly provide assistance to the team as it proceeds on its journey. Familiarity with the tools the team may use is imperative. The facilitator is also responsible for training the team leader and the team in the techniques to be used. Most organizations have to look outside for facilitators, at least until indigenous facilitators can be trained and become experienced.

Teams cannot function in a vacuum; support is vital. First, team members need to understand that the work of the team is not extra work but is considered part of the job. Therefore coverage for team members or allowance for overtime must be arranged. Second, a place to meet and necessary materials must be provided. The location and type of room provided by the leadership speak volumes about the importance, or lack thereof, imparted to team functioning. Third, training must be provided. This may require facilitating the facilitator or seeking support initially from outside the organization, but it must be done. Fourth, implementation of the team's recommendations, the ultimate show of support from leadership, must be assured.

Although the problem statement charging the team with its function may contain conditions, management must be willing to change the process within the team's purview. Constraining conditions imposed on a team may include no new hiring of personnel or spending limits, but clearly conditions that are too intrusive stifle the team. If initial teams are properly and carefully constituted, charged, led, and facilitated and see that recommendations are acted on with dispatch by management, the infectious enthusiasm for the QM approach will be overwhelming. Early concerns about readiness to participate on the part of workers will evaporate as the workers catch on and infect their fellow workers with enthusiasm.

Continuous Quality Improvement

Teams beget teams. As most good scientific inquiries ask more questions than they answer, so do teams identify more processes or parts of processes amenable to team rectification. As well, teams periodically revisit previously enhanced processes to improve them further, and CQI is thus begotten.

Examples of the application of QM techniques in health care may be useful to those contemplating implementation in EMS. Berwick[1] offers a number of illustrative and instructive examples. Because few if any EMS applications of QI are available, the Case Study offers one hospital's experience with a clinically oriented QI project.

Pitfalls of Quality Management

There are pitfalls on the journey to total QM. Some of those pitfalls, drawn from our experience and the literature, are described here. There may be no "buy-in" from top management. Unless the arduous bottom-up incremental implementation approach is contemplated, top management must subscribe. Another pitfall is that the project chosen may be too large. Although in theory there is no project that is too large, initial projects should deliberately be kept small to help ensure success.

The team itself might be problematic. It may include inappropriate members. Team members must know the process and live the process. Although managers, especially middle managers, may be interested and want to become involved, unless they are both knowledgeable of the process under consideration and possessed of the appropriate temperament, they may be inappropriate team members. There may also be a lack of team support. The team needs the space, the time, and the financial support necessary to succeed and will not function as orphans.

There are false prophets abroad in the land; be wary of gurus bearing simple solutions. An organization cannot buy a turnkey solution because too much is dependent on each organization's unique culture for a pat formula to succeed.

Consultants abound who are ready to pounce on those organizations that believe that they can buy a solution or program ready-made.

Impatience can be destructive to implementation of QM. It will take longer than imagined to get started and to see teams perform and results ensue. A project such as that described in the following Case Study may take 4 to 6 months to complete, assuming three to four meetings of 1 hour each per month. Once the team has completed its work, implementation and then reexamination for results must follow, and therefore the entire process from start to assurance of success may take more than 1 year. Although shortcuts may be seductive, there are no shortcuts. QM requires the disciplined application of principles, techniques, and tools, and to attempt shortcuts is to subvert this method of improving quality.

CASE STUDY

The hospital promulgating this QI project is a 179-bed community hospital located in suburban Detroit. The emergency department (ED) attends to approximately 32,000 patients per year. A QA project in the ED showed an opportunity for improvement in the time required to deliver thrombolytic agents to patients for whom such agents were indicated. Coincident with the findings of the QA project was the constitution of a Quality Improvement Council (QIC) at the hospital. The QIC consisted of the medical director and the hospital's CEO, as well as four physicians and four other hospital administrators. One of the physicians on the QIC also served as chief of the ED.

The QIC solicited suggestions for initial QI projects, and one of those selected was based on an apparent need to reduce the time to deliver thrombolytic drugs to ED patients. Among the reasons that this project was chosen were the substantial interest among staff in the emergency center, the project's relatively high profile, the clinical implications, and the ability to be definable, limited, and clear.

The charge to the team was *to examine the process of delivery of thrombolytics to ED patients and to effect a reduction in the time necessary to deliver the drugs.* The QIC identified a team leader and the departments that would probably need to be involved, subject to discussion by the team itself. The CEO of the hospital wrote a letter to the involved department managers requesting nomination of team members.

The team leader identified by the QIC was a staff emergency physician who had an interest in QI techniques. In organizing his team he found that most department managers had nominated participants from the upper echelons of department management. Therefore phone calls were employed to recruit more appropriate members to the team, those who knew the process to be discussed. The facilitator for this team was recruited from the hospital's department of management engineering. This person possessed a superior knowledge of the principles of team functioning, in terms of both group dynamics and tools and techniques. In fact, it was apparent to the QIC that had an indigenous facilitator not been available, training of hospital personnel or recruitment from outside would have been necessary to provide adequate facilitation.

Once the team's composition was set, the team began to meet. The team refined both the problem statement provided by the QIC and the membership of the team suggested by the QIC. This was welcomed by the QIC, as it should be recognized

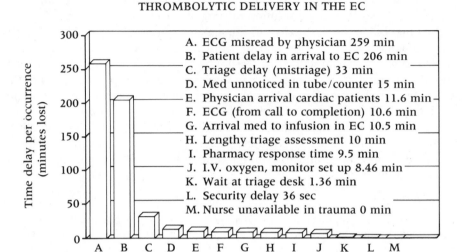

THROMBOLYTIC DELIVERY IN THE EC

A. ECG misread by physician 259 min
B. Patient delay in arrival to EC 206 min
C. Triage delay (mistriage) 33 min
D. Med unnoticed in tube/counter 15 min
E. Physician arrival cardiac patients 11.6 min
F. ECG (from call to completion) 10.6 min
G. Arrival med to infusion in EC 10.5 min
H. Lengthy triage assessment 10 min
I. Pharmacy response time 9.5 min
J. I.V. oxygen, monitor set up 8.46 min
K. Wait at triage desk 1.36 min
L. Security delay 36 sec
M. Nurse unavailable in trauma 0 min

Figure 7-2 Pareto analysis of team data collected in July 1991.

that the people who own the process can best dissect the process. Team membership included representation from emergency physicians, nurses, a registration clerk, an ECG technician, a security officer, a pharmacist, and a cardiologist.

Over the course of approximately 4 months the team went through its diagnostic and remedial journey, using a number of QI techniques (see Figure 7-2 for the Pareto analysis generated). At the same time small problems were identified and rectified when appropriate. Once they understood the process of examining the process, team members became enthusiastic and in fact progressively lengthened their meetings and shortened the intervals between meetings to reach their goal more quickly.

The recommendations of the team have been implemented, with one exception. That exception has resulted in the establishment of a departmental QI team to further examine the process of triage for which no solution was visible to the team examining the administration of thrombolytic agents overall. The thrombolytic team is scheduled to reassemble at intervals to ensure consolidation of gains and to identify further opportunities for improvement.

Each team brings surprises. These surprises emanate both from the dynamics of the team and from the results themselves. This thrombolytic team showed the ED ways to reduce the time of administration of thrombolytics by half. The results of this team's efforts are only the first step. They are now looking for ways to further reduce the time to administer thrombolytics. In the end the problems identified by the team were not those predicted by the ED staff or administration.

Summary

It is said that people do not mind change, they only mind being told to change. QM allows an organization to lead itself at all levels from bottom to top along a path of change. The insights gained from QM at all levels shows an organization along a path toward improved quality. EMS, with its interorganizational structure and often fractious politics, seems ripe for the implementation of QM.

REFERENCES
1. Berwick DM: *Curing health care,* San Francisco, 1990, Jossey-Bass.
2. Deming WE: *Out of crisis.* Cambridge, Mass, 1986, Massachusetts Institute of Technology.
3. Nackel JG, Collier TA: Implementing a quality improvement program, *J Soc Health Syst* 1:85-100, 1989.
4. Sahney VK et al: The process of total quality management in health care, *Frontiers of Health Services Management* 7:2-40, 1991.
5. Scholtes PR: *The team handbook,* Madison, Wis, 1990, Joiner Association.

Section Two

Important Issues in Quality Management

Issues addressed in this section serve as critical building blocks to a successful quality management program. Efforts to improve quality necessitate ready access to data, financial support, and legal protection and recourse to make programs successful. Although these issues are administrative and technical rather than theoretic, ignorance of or inattention to these details can doom attempts to improve quality.

8

Quality Assurance and the Law

Maria B. Abrahamsen, J.D.

Several states have enacted statutes that protect the confidentiality of emergency medical services (EMS) quality assurance (QA) records for the purpose of encouraging candid peer review. A number of states have also adopted laws that provide conditional immunity for QA participants. Such immunity statutes supplement the protection that courts may afford individuals who incidentally harm the reputation or the business interests of another while acting in good faith to protect a public interest. Additionally, practical steps can be taken to enhance the likelihood that QA records qualify for statutory protection of confidentiality and to reduce the risk of liability resulting from participation in QA.

Legal Issues

Two principal legal issues are raised by the performance of QA in any health care setting, including the prehospital arena. The first of these issues is: to what extent can information generated by or for the body that performs QA be kept confidential? Second: what is the potential liability for participants involved in QA activities? These issues are addressed by statute in only a handful of states, and the scope and the nature of statutory protection differ significantly from state to state. By drawing an analogy to the more fully developed law governing QA in the hospital setting, however, it is possible to provide some practical suggestions aimed at protecting the prehospital QA process and its participants.

83

Confidentiality

Reasons for Confidentiality

Those who participate in and those who are the subject of the QA process generally desire to protect QA data from public disclosure, such as release for use in legal proceedings or to the media. Those legislatures and courts that have elected to protect the confidentiality of QA information usually are motivated by an expressed desire to encourage candid QA by assuring the participants that the results will not be made public and may not be used in litigation. In other words, the goal of confidentiality is to protect the integrity of the QA *process* and thereby improve the quality of health care available to the public; the individual *providers* who are the subjects of QA activities are the ancillary beneficiaries of such confidentiality.

On the other hand, strong public policy favors making all relevant information available to the parties involved in litigation, thereby enhancing the likelihood of a just result. Each state attempts to reconcile these conflicting public policies in its statutes and its court decisions relating to the confidentiality of QA records.

State courts are obliged to abide by the QA confidentiality statutes of their state when ruling on the discoverability or admissibility of QA records. However, when federal courts hear lawsuits that are based on federal statutes (such as federal civil rights, antitrust laws, or the Constitution), the federal courts must consider, but are not obliged to follow, state evidenciary laws, including state QA confidentiality statutes.[1]

Confidentiality Statutes

Participants in EMS QA should familiarize themselves with the statute, if any, governing the confidentiality of QA materials in their state. Unless QA materials are made confidential by state statute, they are likely to be subject to subpoena and to other forms of pretrial discovery, and are also admissible as evidence at trial (assuming the materials are relevant and otherwise satisfy generally applicable requirements for the admission of evidence).

EMS QA may be conducted by individual hospitals, individual EMS providers, or a centralized body responsible for the quality of care throughout an EMS. The majority of states have enacted statutes that grant hospital peer-review records at least limited confidentiality. When EMS QA is conducted by a hospital, participants should confirm that the emergency medical care that they review is within the scope of the statutory definition of hospital QA.

Only a handful of states have adopted statutes that expressly make confidential the records of centralized QA conducted by a medical control authority or other body responsible for reviewing the care provided by multiple prehospital providers.[2] For example, the Oregon legislature[3] has expressly provided that "written reports, notes or records" of "any committee or governing body which has the authority to undertake an evaluation of an emergency medical service system as part of a quality assurance program" shall not be deemed public records nor be admissible in evidence in any judicial proceeding. The same Oregon statute provides that persons who serve on or communicate information to such a governing body or committee may not be examined (e.g., deposed or required to testify at trial) regarding communications to the QA body or its findings.

A larger number of states protect the confidentiality of QA conducted by a single EMS provider with respect to its own services.[4] It is unclear, however, whether such confidentiality statutes cover QA conducted on a centralized basis, such as when a committee consisting of representatives of the local medical control authority performs QA. In states that protect only the records of individual providers, QA participants might attempt to bring themselves within the statute's protection by having each provider sign a simple form delegating its QA functions to the centralized medical control committee. Although this approach has not been tested in any reported decision, there is strong appeal to the theory that if QA is confidential when conducted by individual providers, it should also be protected when performed (perhaps more effectively and efficiently) on a centralized basis by a group of providers.

Peer review confidentiality statutes also differ with respect to the scope of confidentiality created by each. The principal variables include:

- Type of information protected: data submitted to the QA body, the body's deliberations and/or its conclusions; written records only; or also prohibition against requiring participants to testify.
- Type of QA protected: prospective (such as development of protocols and policies); concurrent; and/or retrospective.
- Whose records are protected: specified bodies only; or any individual and/or body that performs a QA function.
- Protection from what: pretrial discovery; and/or admission as evidence at trial.
- Absolute prohibition against disclosure or a "privilege" that may be waived by the provider who is the subject of review and/or the QA body. If the former, the statute may either prohibit the use of QA information in *all* proceedings or only in professional liability actions and/or other types of personal-injury lawsuits against providers.

Participants in EMS QA can be effective advocates for confidentiality legislation that incorporates broad protection with respect to each of the variables outlined above.

Practical Steps to Enhance Confidentiality

Although the measures that enhance the confidentiality of QA records vary from state to state and depend on the state's specific statute and case law, the following general considerations are relevant in all jurisdictions:

What are the defined elements of QA?   The bylaws and procedures of individual prehospital providers and of medical control bodies should expressly designate those committees and individuals who are responsible for QA, such as the medical control authority's chief medical officer, QA committee, and governing body. Bylaws and procedures should also describe each QA function as constituting "peer review" or whatever other terminology the applicable state statute uses to define confidential records. A court is more apt to respect the confidentiality of QA materials if there is evidence that a clearly organized QA system exists.

By whom are QA data collected and analyzed?   QA data should be collected and analyzed solely by individuals or committees who have been formally assigned a QA function, as described in the preceding paragraph. If, for example, providers are asked to prepare summaries or incident reports that will be used in QA, QA policies should state that these documents constitute QA materials. Access to the documents should then be limited to formally designated QA participants.

The importance of clearly defining what constitutes QA data is illustrated by two court decisions that arose under a statute[8] that makes confidential the "data and records collected by or for an individual or committee" granted a hospital peer-review duty. In one ruling the court held that this statute did not protect data that were collected independently by a physician and later turned over to a hospital QA committee.[5] The court based its decision on the fact that the data were not *initially* gathered at the behest of a person or committee assigned a QA function. However, in another case interpreting the same statute the court held that hospital incident reports constitute confidential QA materials that could not be subpoenaed, based on evidence that the reports were generated for the purpose of reducing morbidity and mortality, and pursuant to hospital policy the reports were submitted to the hospital's safety and/or QA committees.[6]

In short the likelihood that data can be kept confidential is significantly enhanced if the QA body identifies prospectively the types of data that are considered confidential and if access to such data is limited to those who have been formally granted QA duties.

How are QA records maintained and distributed?   As a general rule, courts are willing to protect QA records from public disclosure only if the health care provider holding the records has also respected the confidentiality of the records. For example, a court does not look with sympathy on a request that QA committee minutes be protected from subpoena if the minutes have been widely distributed prior to receipt of the subpoena. All documents generated by a QA body that the participants hope to protect (such as QA committee minutes and reports) should be appropriately marked (e.g., with the notation "Confidential/ Peer Review Materials"). The terminology chosen for the notation should conform with the language of the state's confidentiality statute. Some providers photocopy each page of QA materials onto special paper that contains such a notation.

It is also wise to identify patients and providers by number, rather than by name, in QA documents. This practice reduces the risk of harm to an individual's reputation in the event the documents are circulated inappropriately.

If the QA committee is required to report its activities or findings to other bodies that are not clearly covered by a peer-review confidentiality statute, the committee's reports should be concise and should not contain information that the committee wishes to protect against subpoena or other public disclosure. Particular care should be taken when releasing QA information to public bodies, such as county and state agencies, since records in the possession of public bodies are frequently subject to public disclosure under a state freedom-of-information act, unless protected by a specific exemption.

To reduce the chance that the QA records will be inappropriately distributed and the privileged nature of such records waived, it is good practice to collect copies of all QA materials at the end of QA committee meetings unless it is essential that members retain such materials. Responsibility for maintaining QA records should be centralized and access limited to those who have a legitimate QA function to perform. It is preferable if access to confidential records is governed by a written policy.

Liability

Types of Potential Liability

Individuals who submit information to an EMS QA body, and its members, frequently express concern regarding the potential for liability as a result of their participation in QA. The following types of claims are the most likely to arise as a result of QA:

1. A defamation (libel or slander) claim by the provider who is the subject of review, particularly if QA information regarding the provider is disclosed in a manner contrary to a confidentiality statute. A successful defamation claim requires evidence that the defendant, knowing that the information was false or at least negligently failing to ascertain the facts, transmitted to a third party false information regarding the plaintiff that harmed the plaintiff's reputation.

2. An antitrust claim and/or claim of tortious interference with business relationships by a provider who experienced licensure discipline and/or adverse publicity as a result of QA; for example, a claim that competing providers conspired to eliminate the plaintiff from the market or to secure the plaintiff's customers for themselves.

3. A claim by a patient who was injured while receiving EMS that QA was performed negligently, resulting in proper protocols not being in place or an incompetent provider being permitted to continue to practice.

Immunity Statutes

To encourage candid participation in the QA process a number of states have enacted statutes that provide immunity from liability arising from the performance of QA.[7]

In addition, the federal Health Care Quality Improvement Act of 1986 (42 U.S.C. §§11101-11152) creates qualified immunity for the participants in certain forms of peer review. This federal statute is unlikely, however, to provide immunity for EMS QA activities because (1) it protects only against claims brought by physicians (defined as M.D., D.O., and D.D.S.); (2) it covers only professional review actions of a "health care entity," which is defined as being an entity that both provides health care (or is a professional society) and follows a formal peer-review process; and (3) it covers only actions that adversely affect a physician's clinical privileges or membership in a health care entity.

The principal variables among immunity statutes include:

- Persons covered: members of a QA body, those who furnish information to a QA body, those who investigate on behalf of or otherwise counsel or assist a QA body, and/or the body itself.
- Prerequisites to immunity: no malice, good faith, and/or reasonable belief that action was warranted by facts known.
- Types of claims protected against: claims for monetary damages only, all civil claims, or all civil and criminal claims.

Immunity statutes do not preclude a plaintiff from filing a lawsuit against QA participants. The existence of an immunity statute does not even necessarily ensure that a lawsuit is dismissed at an early stage (e.g., on motion for summary judgment), since there may be factual disputes as to whether the defendants satisfy the statutory requirements for immunity. However, immunity statutes increase the number of facts the plaintiff must prove to succeed in his lawsuit; for example, the existence of an immunity statute might require the plaintiff to prove that the defendants acted in bad faith while participating in QA.

Common-Law Protection

In addition to specific immunity statutes, the courts have developed certain principles that protect against liability in cases alleging defamation of character or interference with business relationships. There is common-law protection (or, in legal parlance, a privilege) against defamation liability for communications made in good faith and in the reasonable belief that the communication was necessary to fulfill a moral or legal duty, provided the disclosure is limited to appropriate individuals and to proper subject matter.

Similarly, if a person acts to protect a public interest or for other laudable purposes, he may be protected by the courts from a claim of interference with business relationships, especially if the defendants' actions were not unreasonable in light of the threatened harm. Common-law privileges of this sort generally are not well defined and are highly dependent on the facts of each case. Nevertheless, when QA participants act reasonably for the purpose of improving public health care and are not motivated by self-interest, they may be protected from liability by common-law privileges.

Practical Steps to Reduce Risk of Liability

The risk that those who conduct EMS QA or those who furnish information to a QA body will incur liability as a result of such participation can be reduced by taking the following measures:

Follow the QA body's own bylaws and procedures. This enhances the likelihood that review activities will be deemed part of official QA and therefore qualify for any available immunity and/or privilege.

Do not permit the QA process to be misused. QA participants should diligently avoid use of the QA process for any purpose other than improvement of patient care. To prevent even the appearance that QA is being used to further the financial interests of participants, try to avoid having providers participate in decisions from which they might benefit.

Preserve the confidentiality of the QA records. By doing so, the QA body reduces the risk that the reputation of a provider who is the subject of review will be harmed, thereby also reducing risk of a successful claim of defamation or interference with business relationships.

Summary

Participants in EMS QA should familiarize themselves with the laws of their state regarding confidentiality of QA materials and immunity from liability for QA participants. If the QA confidentiality and/or the immunity statutes have been interpreted by state courts (whether in the context of QA conducted by an EMS organization or any other type of health care provider), QA participants should also be familiar with these rulings. The policies, minutes, reports, and other documents of the QA body should be drafted in a manner that maximizes the likelihood that confidentiality and immunity will apply to their QA activities. All QA activities should be conducted with consideration for the consequences to confidentiality and to immunity. QA participants in states that do not presently have QA confidentiality or immunity statutes covering EMS QA should consider seeking enactment of such statutes.

REFERENCES

1. *See, e.g.,* Dorsten v. Lapeer County General Hospital, 88 F.R.D. 583 (E.D. Mich. 1980) and Robinson v. Magovern, 83 F.R.D. 79 (W.D. Pa. 1979).
2. Ga. Code Ann. §31-7-131, as construed in Op. Atty. Gen. 88-5 (Jan. 27, 1988); 1989 Or. Laws, ch. 1079; Fla. Stat. §401.425; Wash. Rev. Code §70.168.090 (1990).
3. 1989 Or. Laws, ch. 1079.
4. *See, e.g.,* Mich. Comp. Laws Ann. §351.531 *et seq.* and §333.20175(6); Nev. Rev. Stat. §49.265; Tex. Gen. Laws 605 (§773.095).
5. Marchand v. Henry Ford Hospital, 398 Mich. 163, 247 N.W.2d 280 (1976).

6. Gallagher v. Detroit-Macomb Hospital Association, 171 Mich. App. 761 (1988).
7. *See, e.g.,* Fla. Stat. §401.425; Ga. Code Ann. §331-7-132; Mich. Comp. Laws Ann. §331.531, *et seq.*; 1989 Or. Laws, ch. 1079; and 1991 Tex. Gen. Laws 605 (§773.096).
8. Mich. Comp. Laws §333.21515.

9

Data Collection and Management

Ameen I. Ramzy, M.D.
John New, B.A.

"Data" are defined as factual information used as a basis for reasoning, discussion, or calculation. Data collection and management in emergency medical services (EMS) constitutes one of the potentially most tedious and demanding, yet valuable, components of quality assurance (QA). As a measure of the effectiveness of EMS, data collection must yield uniform information. This uniformity allows comparisons within and among systems and thus is an appropriate and necessary step in the QA process.

The public today not only respects the people and processes that deliver EMS but also *expects* efficient and effective emergency response and treatment when injury or illness occurs. The modern medical world offers antisepsis, anesthesia, and antibiotics, as well as sophisticated radiologic imaging techniques, emergency cardiac care, and trauma-EMS systems. These diagnostic and therapeutic measures have developed only recently. In previous centuries, injured and ill people may have fared better without being subjected to some of the medicinal and surgical practices of the times.

Now, however, high expectations for the delivery of lifesaving and restorative medical care vie with concern about health-care costs, questions regarding access to care, and a litigious milieu. Those in EMS systems, therefore, must seek and develop tools that ensure that EMS care is of the highest possible quality. Progress toward this goal is measured through data collection and success in access and interpretation of valid and reliable data.

Concepts in Data Collection

The ideal data collection process is painless, inexpensive, and manageable. Unfortunately, such a data collection process does not yet exist, especially for large systems. Several approaches and methods do exist, however, and these are reviewed along with their advantages and disadvantages.

Physicians are most familiar with the narrative medical record because most patient medical records are kept in this fashion. Since a patient may be treated by many medical care providers for the same illness over a period spanning his lifetime, each person administering care is obligated to record relevant information for those who may follow. In the conventional documentation approach, physicians record a patient's history through handwritten daily progress notes and dictated and transcribed discharge summaries (the primary data source). An additional type of record collection is a "registry;" examples include tumor registries and trauma registries. Information for such records is usually based on a patient's written history, abstracted by data collectors, and accessed by physicians only in its completed form.

The prehospital record (also known as a "run sheet" or "prehospital care record") has the primary goal of documenting the care provided to an individual patient from the injury or illness scene to a hospital or during interfacility transport. A secondary, but important, function of the record is to serve as an EMS system assessment tool. This "double tasking" of prehospital records must be taken into consideration during the planning of such record-keeping processes.

The EMS record of the future may be very different. Perhaps in the not-too-distant future the prehospital field provider will "think out loud" into a headset. The audio signal will then be transmitted to a computer that will not only transcribe the information but also collate it into an individual medical record that is printed at the receiving hospital. This record will provide hospital clinicians with timely, uniform assessment data to anticipate the patient's needs and allow them to be ready when the patient and prehospital-care provider arrive at the hospital. The EMS care provider can review, correct, and sign the document while a separate system record is being collated and automatically transcribed.

Although such technology is not farfetched, it is cost-prohibitive at present. Even when the technology is commonly available and economically feasible, writing and signing an individual record remains valuable because of the discipline, individual responsibility, and accountability involved.[4] When prehospital-care providers record on-scene times, awareness of critical time aspects of prehospital care is heightened.

The EMS record should measure the demand or request for service, the response to that request, and the outcome (Table 9-1). These three elements should be measured both for the individual patient and for the total EMS system. The definition of the EMS system response can be local (squad, municipality, or county), statewide, or cover a multistate region. This "multitasking" of the EMS record, again, reflects the dual responsibility and value of EMS records for the

Table 9-1. EMS Record Considerations by Function

Question objectives	Medical record Specific goals	Data considerations
1. Who was treated?	A. Patient identifiers	Patient name Patient address Residence co/city Residence state Residence zip code
	B. Associated patient information	Guardian Telephone number Residence type
	C. Incident identifier	Incident number Incident location Call number Local information
2. What was known about the patient's condition?	D. Patient history	Preexisting conditions Medications Allergies
	E. Patient assessment	Chief complaint Narrative description
3. What was the course of care?	F. Documentation of care rendered	Interventions by provider ID/ Time/vitals/rhythm/care/ amount
	G. Documentation of care refused	IV therapy Services Services & transport
4. Who were the responsible parties involved with patient care?	H. Prehospital	Driver's name/ID number Attendant's name (2)/ID number Form completed by signature Other(s) on scene
	I. Hospital	Patient received by signature
5. What was the outcome of prehospital care?	J. Outcome after transport	ED vitals ED diagnosis ED disposition ED death date and time

Continued.

Table 9-1. EMS Record Considerations by Function—cont'd

Question objectives	System assessment Specific goals	Data considerations
1. What requests/demands were made of EMS?	A. Identify request types	Signs/symptoms Injury type Medical conditions
	B. Acuity assessment	Priority status First vital signs Unconsciousness (prior to arrival) ECG Cardiac arrest Glasgow coma score Trauma identification Mechanisms
	C. Information related to person	Patient age Patient race Patient gender
	D. Information related to time	Time of 9-1-1 call Time of ambulance call Transport month, day, & year
	E. Information related to place	Census tract number
2. What was the response to the request?	F. Identify who and special circumstances of response	Unit county Unit number Dispatch status First due status No care rendered options Safety equipment Special purpose
	G. Assess sequence of response	Time of station departure Time of location arrival Time of location departure Time of hospital arrival Time of return to service
	H. Record intervention	Management Oxygen Airway IV Medications
	I. Account for unit staffing	Highest certified level

Continued.

Table 9-1. EMS Record Considerations by Function—cont'd

Question objectives	System assessment Specific goals	Data considerations
3. What was the outcome?	J. Disposition after assessment	Transport status Transfer reasons
	K. Communications	Consulting hospital Radio quality
	L. Facility demand	Transferring hospital Receiving hospital
	M. Facility determination	Reason hospital chosen
	N. Form review	EMS reviewer signature
4. What flexibility exists for future data needs?	O. Self-defined data	Generic data field

individual patient and for the EMS system. Although this three-phase recording of demand, response, and outcome is conceptually simple if not intuitive, it is the cornerstone for record design and implementation.

Although there is no national uniformity as to precise EMS data elements, recent proposals have been made. Hedges and Joyce[2] describe 20 data elements to be included in EMS reports. Portions of their recommendations are derived from the Maryland Ambulance Information System (MAIS) (Figure 9-1).[1] Currently, the National Highway Traffic Safety Administration is developing a consensus-defined minimum EMS data set. This project is attempting to standardize definitions and to facilitate uniform reporting of prehospital-care data.

Methods of Data Collection

Although the three basic areas that EMS records should measure are clear, opinions vary as to how the EMS data system should collect and measure that information. At present the options range from pure narrative to structured narrative to pure optical scanning. In the future, technology will become available to allow for reliable computer imaging of handwritten information. To date, this process is an expensive proposition with untested measures of feasibility and accuracy. This discussion focuses on the narrative and optical-scanning approaches, considering their advantages and disadvantages.

A pure narrative record offers the advantage of being most useful to the clinician receiving patients. The richness of detail that a properly written narrative allows conveys considerable information that confirms and supple-

Figure 9-1 (part 1) The MAIS form serves as a medical record of care and a collection of system-assessment data elements. It represents information standardized in content and definition. (From Maryland Institute for Emergency Medical Services Systems.)

ments voice or face-to-face communications between the prehospital-care provider and the receiving physician. The disadvantages of a pure narrative record are the potential variability in what is recorded, the legibility of the handwriting, and the prohibitive cost to individually abstract every narrative record for EMS system data collection.

A variant of the pure narrative is a structured narrative in which the prehospital-care provider records information in specific categories or completes a checklist of structured responses. Such information may lose a little of the specific detail of a pure narrative, but it provides an objective means by which all responses can be categorized. This type of run sheet is often quicker and easier to complete in the field. It also facilitates data abstraction by a technique such as keypunching.

Pure optical scanning offers the advantage of theoretic consistency of data entry, which is important when dealing with large numbers of EMS responses. This process has the disadvantage of making it more difficult for the clinician receiving the patient to process such information from a scan sheet as opposed to a written narrative. Another limitation of optical scanning is that it predefines categories of information and thus may preclude subtleties of clinical information that need to be conveyed through either verbal communication or additional narrative.

At the present time a blend of narrative and optical scanning is the preferred method. This is not simply a compromise but a recognition that the EMS report is a record of the care rendered to an individual patient *and* an EMS system assessment tool.

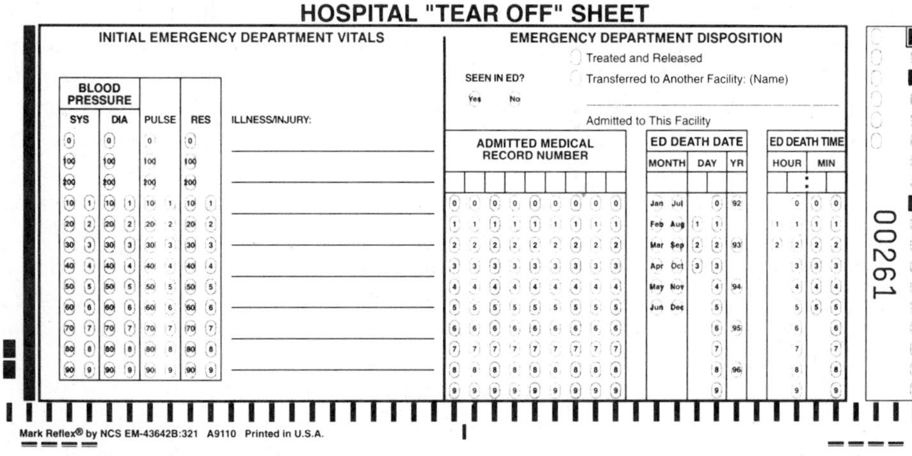

Figure 9-1 (part 2) The MAIS form serves as a medical record of care and a collection of system-assessment data elements. It represents information standardized in content and definition.

Initiating a Data Collection System

For EMS systems that do not yet have a standard run sheet there are several ways to get started. Perhaps the most disadvantageous way is to select a vendor to print run sheets, to select the data points, and to distribute them. Such an approach is less likely to yield positive results because the informational content of a record should not drive the informational need.

A far more prudent way is to first decide what the EMS system wants the run sheet to do. In other words a run sheet is not a goal or an end in itself; it is merely a means to a goal. The goal is to measure request, response, and outcome. A particular EMS system may articulate its goals in another way. For example, the goal of a trauma system, as a subset of the EMS system, may be the eradication of preventable death and disability as a result of trauma.[3]

The process of developing an EMS report for a given area depends on leadership and consensus building. The EMS community must be involved. The very definition of "EMS community" engenders discussion. A potential definition should include prehospital-care providers, EMS supervisors, jurisdictional authorities, regional managers, receiving physicians and hospitals, EMS planners and evaluators, EMS organizations, and the state EMS program office.

A three-phase process should be considered in EMS report development. The first phase is to articulate the questions the report should be capable of answering and to identify routine reports that provide meaningful answers. The second phase is to select and to approve the record's structure. The third phase is to draft pilot tests and implement the report. Many general and specific issues arise in such a process. The following discussion is not intended to provide the answers to these issues but to aid in anticipating them.

The format of the report raises a number of issues and decision points. First, will the report be one or two pages? For receiving clinicians and system managers, the more information the better. However, for the prehospital-care provider completing the EMS report, there must be realism and practicality. Since all calls involve primarily basic life support (BLS) and the majority require no higher level of care, should one report be used for BLS calls and a separate one for advanced life support (ALS) calls? Although such an approach may be appealing, it can indeed be cumbersome. In some systems ALS units may respond and provide strictly BLS care. In other circumstances a BLS unit may respond and provide all the patient's care because of the logistics of ALS response. Therefore we recommend a single EMS report form for both BLS and ALS responses. We have also found that a majority of calls can be reported accurately on a single page, with an optional second page for additional narrative or billing information.

The second consideration concerning format is the actual size of the report. Both standard-size (8½ × 11 inches) and legal-size (8½ × 14 inches) report forms were introduced and used in Maryland. Ultimately, the legal size, although offering more room for information documentation, was found to be cumbersome by the prehospital-care provider and more susceptible to damage. Forms that were torn or bent at the edges impeded the efficiency of centralized scanning.

A third issue relates to the narrative and the optically scanned information. Unfortunately, no "prescription" predefines this. This is one of the issues that the EMS community has to work through and make a judgment as to what information is most necessary to meet both the needs of the individual patient's record (and thus be narrative oriented) and those of the EMS system (represented by optical mark responses).

An additional format issue is to create a layout of the run sheet that provides a logical flow of information. If the information flow on the sheet parallels the way a prehospital-care provider approaches an incident response and patient care, records the information, and relays that information by radio, the entire documentation process is more successful in terms of accuracy and compliance.

Another format consideration is the number of copies required. This again varies according to the local system. In most situations either three or four copies are necessary. One copy remains at the receiving facility with the patient as a document of patient history and care, becoming part of the patient's permanent chart; one copy goes to a data collection center for central data submission purposes; and at least one additional copy stays with the local prehospital-care provider organization (i.e., ambulance unit or station) as the official record and basis for the QA review. In some EMS services an additional copy goes to the central office of the ambulance service to be used as an additional QA-review procedure.

Other important logistic considerations include the training of EMS personnel to use the forms, the centralization or decentralization of the data collection process, and the type of reports to be generated from the information. Like any other aspect of health care or EMS, an innovation requires training and familiarization. When an EMS report is introduced into a system, training in its use should cover the following: the purpose of the form, the content, the explanation of variables and appropriate responses, and the procedures for completing the form and submitting it to the data processing center. The resources for conducting and evaluating training sessions must also be identified.

The question of centralized or decentralized data processing must also be addressed. The advantages of both systems are compared in Table 9-2. Although it may be appealing to enter data locally and then transmit it to a central processing area, tremendous resources can be expended (successfully and sometimes unsuccessfully) in electronic linkage systems. The most reliable process is to ensure that a hard copy of the EMS report gets to a central processing center. We do not recommend using regular mail service for such important documents; in Maryland, regional EMS administrators are responsible for form collection and delivery to the central processing department.

The aggregate reports to be generated from individual run sheets must be anticipated. The types and timing of reports should be defined in advance using the same process that developed the EMS run sheet for the community. For example, municipalities or regions may request detailed information on types of calls or response times. The report format should answer the initial consideration: what questions should my instrument be capable of answering? Tailoring reports to specific needs and requests is preferable to a "shotgun" approach in which virtually every piece of information is automatically reported back to the

Table 9-2. Advantages of Centralized vs. Decentralized Data Collection

Centralized	Decentralized
1. More cost-effective a. Single processing center (hardware, software, staff)	1. Faster access to local information

2. Better standardization of information	2. Better editing procedures
	    a. Closer to the source
	    b. Vested interest

3. More consistent process management	3. Potentially better ad hoc analysis capabilities

EMS agency transporting the patient. If reports are not tailored, then reams of computer printouts masking valuable information are generated, distributed, and ignored.

Access to information must be considered in advance. One approach is to include the hospital copy of the EMS report as part of the hospital medical record. The official record is the copy maintained by the EMS service, whereas the data-collection copy may be considered a statistical record only. In this way requests for copies of the record can be correctly referred to the prehospital EMS service that provided the care. Keep in mind that all policies for patient confidentiality and access to records must comply with state law.

Data collection and management costs must be anticipated prior to instituting the process. Hardware, software, and maintenance must be considered in addition to the actual costs of printing run sheets. Even more important are costs associated with data entry, editing, and analysis, as well as financing the EMS program's management.

If optical scanning is used, the steps involved in processing must be appreciated. This presumes that the logistics of collecting forms at a central location have already been met. Once the forms are collected they must be reviewed individually to ensure "scanability" (removal of any staples and erasure of stray marks) and to verify jurisdictional codes for valid batch processing. Forms are then batch-fed through a scanner at a rate of approximately 700 per hour. (Scanning rates of 5000 plus per hour are available at considerable costs.) A computer language file (ASCII) is then written to a transfer medium, which is customarily tape because of the volume of the data that must be carried. The tapes are transferred to a management environment, which in our situation is a VAX 11/780. Central files are then edited for processing and archived to main storage. Reports are generated based on protocols. Individual forms are then microfiched and reviewed for image quality before confidential disposal of any run sheets. State law often dictates the period of time patient records must be kept.

Our 8 years of experience with optically scanned and narrative run sheets have been favorable. We are currently revising our run sheet data points, using the process previously described, to make the run sheets of greater value, particularly with the addition of outcome measures. Table 9-3 provides an inventory of the costs associated with processing approximately 300,000 forms annually in Maryland.

Although EMS reports are a primary data collection mechanism in QA, other data bases should also be considered. Approximately half the states in the United States (and five of the seven mid-Atlantic states) use hospital discharge-reporting data sets. These indicate total hospital discharges and list from 5 to 15 diagnoses per patient. They are valuable data bases for population-based studies. A number of states and areas also have specialty-care registries, such as trauma registries. These are often hospital-based rather than population-based, but serve a specific value. Other data bases, including the state motor vehicle accidents report and fire incident casualty report, may also be beneficial.

Table 9-3. Examples of Maryland's Optical Scanning Operating Costs Based on 300,000 Forms Processed per Year

	Dollars
Initial costs	
Optical scanner rated at 700 forms/hr	$6855
(Includes ScanTools software, installation, and automatic sheet-feeding option)	
Development of proof(s) and final form	800
Tape drive	2250
Personal computer and monochrome monitor	1500
(Tape device port card included)	
Microfiche reader/printer	1625
(lenses included)	
Continued annual costs	
Printing of optical scan forms (400,000)	51,900
Personnel	44,000
(1.0 Data processing programmer; 0.5 data processing data entry operator)	
Archival storage	7600
(Microfiche copy paper included)	
Hardware maintenance	1684
(Scanner, tape drive, and microfiche viewer)	
Coping of quarterly and annual reports	1643
(43,800 pages at 3.75 cents per copy)	
Mass data storage	1000
(1 Removable disk, 2 dozen tapes)	
Variable cost*	
Central computer processing	0-40,000
(Disk storage, connect time, and CPU time)	

*Varies according to locally available computer access.

Summary

EMS data collection must be tailored to the specific goals of the EMS system. Data collection, performed either manually or through computer assistance, should measure EMS requests, response, and patient outcome. Selected outcome measures are the most difficult information to capture but yield the most comprehensive data collection instrument.

REFERENCES

1. Bell JM et al: Computer management of prehospital information, *J Emerg Med Serv* 7(12):33-38, 1982.
2. Hedges JR, Joyce SM: Minimum data set for EMS report form: historical development and future implications, *Prehosp Disaster Med* 5(4):383-388, 1990.
3. Ramzy A: A new agenda for trauma, *Am Coll Surg Bull* 72(9):10-11, 26, 1987.
4. Spaite DW et al: A prospective evaluation of prehospital patient assessment by direct in-field observation: failure of ALS personnel to measure vital signs, *Prehosp Disaster Med* 5(4):325-334, 1990.

ACKNOWLEDGMENT

The authors appreciate the assistance of Marjorie Enko and Linda Kesselring in the preparation of this chapter.

10

Discipline in Prehospital Emergency Medical Care

Garry Briese, CAE
Robert Pringle, Jr., NREMT-P

The field of prehospital emergency medical care is dynamic and therefore requires careful, constant monitoring to ensure consistent high-quality patient care. In addition, emergency medical services (EMS) providers must conduct themselves in a highly self-disciplined manner. Yet despite such high patient care standards, performance and discipline problems do develop.

Problems in prehospital EMS typically "result from poor job design (overly complex systems), training inadequacies, failure of leadership, or an unclear purpose."[1] Since medical directors provide the operational framework and authorization for paramedics and emergency medical technicians (EMTs), it is imperative that physicians understand and become intimately involved in the development and implementation of EMS disciplinary policy.

Quality Assurance and Discipline

Can a quality assurance (QA) program be integrated with a disciplinary program? The answer is a resounding *yes*. Although the goal of both programs is to increase performance level of quality patient care, it must be kept in mind that all actions must be corrective, not punitive, in nature. Regrettably, many field providers equate QA activities with discipline. This is certainly not the intent, and the very need for disciplinary procedures suggests that the QA process itself has failed—that care has not been improved by documenting an issue and identifying it for the individuals or the area involved. Virtually every method of QA outlined in previous chapters has stressed an educational, supportive approach to improvement of care. Only when all other methods have failed and the provider is resistant to reasonable efforts to change should the disciplinary process be invoked.

EMS Discipline Problems

Paramedic or EMT discipline is an awkward subject for most medical directors, since discipline is a subject largely ignored in the EMS literature. Yet more and more medical directors are finding themselves faced with the reality of disciplining a member of the prehospital team.

The three major problems in EMS discipline are as follows:

1. *The lack of specific procedures for handling discipline situations.* Many EMS systems still have not developed procedures for handling difficult performance situations. This is especially true in third-service EMS systems, volunteer EMS organizations, private companies, and in the less structured environment of nonunionized EMS organizations.
2. *The lack of training managers and medical directors have handling discipline situations.* When asked, most medical directors feel that disciplining an EMS team member is perhaps the most difficult part of their job. If the EMS departments or organizations do not have well-documented written procedures to handle discipline situations, the difficulty of each situation is further compounded by the lack of training given to medical directors. This results in an ad hoc or improvised approach to discipline, which in turn makes both the medical director and the EMS provider unhappy with the process and the result.
3. *The lack of training for EMTs and paramedics in their role in the discipline process.* Just as managers must be trained how to initiate and to manage the discipline process, so must EMS personnel be trained for their role in that process. For example, if EMTs and paramedics are not given feedback on how to improve or to correct their performance, they cannot complete their role in the disciplinary process. The EMT or paramedic must be knowledgeable of the process to accept the discipline.

In the Beginning

To reduce the need for a lengthy disciplinary action, supervisors and physicians must make every effort to educate and train personnel thoroughly in every aspect of expected conduct and performance.[6] This includes documenting that all personnel have read the policy and the procedure documents. Often, simply bringing the problem to the attention of the provider resolves the situation. Once notified, however, it becomes the employee's responsibility to modify his performance in accordance with the policy.

If a more serious problem in job performance is discovered, it must be decided to solve the problem through:

1. Training
2. Employee assistance services

3. Nondisciplinary counseling or
4. Disciplinary action

Within the Phoenix Fire Department each situation is considered separately, making the supervisor responsible for determining the best course of action to take to resolve the situation.[5] In some systems the physician may be solely responsible for this determination or may act in conjunction with agency supervisors. Adhering to a guideline that similar situations receive similar attention and course of action prevents the impression of arbitrariness or impropriety.

Discipline Objectives

The principal objective of any disciplinary policy and subsequent action must be to improve or to correct performance, efficiency, and morale of the individual, and to improve these characteristics in the EMS organization or the department through individual actions. The policy must therefore be administered "in a corrective, progressive and lawful manner."[5]

Types of Discipline

Corrective discipline implies that the medical director understands the causes and the reasons for the deficiency. He must work to correct the problem and to restore the prehospital-care provider to a productive and positive status.

Progressive discipline incorporates several levels of action to be taken. Disciplinary action for an individual normally begins with a verbal reprimand or warning. If subsequent incidents (related or not) warrant action, then disciplinary action should proceed to a written reprimand, suspension without pay, demotion, and finally dismissal. An incident of nonadherence to the policies of the agency or the department may require that any or all these forms of action be taken, regardless of whether a lesser form of disciplinary action has preceded the current action. This of course depends on the severity of the offense.

Finally, discipline must be carried out in a lawful manner. The action to be taken cannot violate personnel rules of the jurisdiction, administrative procedure acts, rules of conduct, labor-management agreements, standard operating procedures, or constitutional rights of the individual. With this in mind, the medical director must know the organization's or the department's policy concerning confidentiality. Normally, the proceedings from disciplinary hearings and the results are held confidential.

An excellent example of mandating a need for confidentiality is the Kenosha County, Wis., EMS policy concerning disputes in medical treatment. It simply states: "All system participants that are parties to a dispute . . . are forbidden from discussing the dispute outside of the presence of the Paramedic EMS Coordinator and the Co-Project Medical Directors," and all proceedings and information must be maintained in complete confidence.[2] The policy continues by imposing a penalty of "disciplinary action" for disclosure of confidential information. It is therefore incumbent upon the physician to maintain this confidentiality.

Effect of Quality Assurance on Discipline

As previously mentioned, both QA and discipline programs strive for quality patient care. If a QA program steps outside of the realm of corrective action, the entire program could very well be in jeopardy. EMTs and paramedics are like all other professionals in medicine: if continuous disciplinary action results from a QA program, they will inevitably protect themselves from further action by "covering" themselves. Although the QA program may view the problem as being resolved, it may still exist or even become worse.

Thus the need to prevent QA issues from always representing discipline becomes apparent. If medical directors and managers of EMS agencies strive for a QA program to be a team approach and prevent it from becoming continuously punitive in nature, the entire problem can be avoided. By making both programs corrective, support for the programs will build, making the goal of quality patient care easily attainable.

Variables

The medical director should always consult with the offender's supervisor or chief to ensure support prior to taking disciplinary action. The physician must also be confident that the actions can be supported in a formal review or an appeal process. The disciplinary actions should be reviewed by nonmedical superiors and be subject to grievance processes or civil service appeals.[5]

Physicians involved in the direction of EMS systems in which labor unions are present must keep in mind that employees have the right to union representation throughout the disciplinary process, if they so choose. Depending on the system, the individual may request not to be represented by his union. If this is a permissible action in the organization, the request should be honored and documented.

If the individual being disciplined is alleged to have committed a criminal act, he may request legal representation during disciplinary proceedings. The counsel's role should be limited to advising the individual, not to answering questions.

Retraining

If the problem is determined to be due to a deficit in the provider's training, an individual program of improvement, not discipline, should be developed. In developing this program the physician must first clearly define the performance problem area(s) and incorporate measurable objectives for continued improvement. To be fair and just to the provider the program must indicate a reasonable time frame in which the objectives must be met.

An essential aspect of the improvement program is the documentation of the provider's status at the end of the period. If an individual has not shown sufficient improvement as measured by the objectives, the situation should be dealt with as a disciplinary problem.

Allegations

Any accusation of misconduct or complaint received from a credible source should be investigated. This information may also be obtained from medical audits by supervisors, medical directors, or other providers. The investigation must be initiated *before* formal action is taken. It must be stressed to all involved that the investigation is a fact-finding process. Supervisors and medical directors must be cautioned not to make statements or judgments until a thorough investigation has been concluded. Depending on the department or organization, the medical director or the chief of the department, with the approval of the city/county manager, may have the discretion to suspend with pay or to reassign the provider pending the outcome of the investigation.

If permissible by the system the medical director may immediately suspend a prehospital-care provider if he believes that immediate suspension (with pay) is necessary to ensure the public's health and safety.[4] This action should only be taken if it is warranted by the seriousness of the alleged infraction. In addition, the state certifying agency should be notified of the suspension.

Investigations

The methods of investigation are as varied as the EMS systems themselves. The process is generally performed by the agency or the organization that employs the individual. In most cases the medical director is asked to assist in the investigation, but the extent of involvement depends on the standard operating procedures and policies of the jurisdiction.

Once a thorough investigation into an incident or complaint has been completed and the need for disciplinary action has been determined, the medical director (in conjunction with the individual's supervisors) must make a decision concerning the most effective action to be taken. In making this decision several factors should be considered:

1. The seriousness of the offense
2. The individual's past history
3. Past practice of the agency in dealing with similar offenses
4. Consistency is critical

Making It Work

Of the previously listed factors, consistency is the most imperative; without it, an effective disciplinary system cannot exist. Although disciplinary actions for the same offenses should be similar, the final decision to determine the exact action should only be made after considering the above factors and applying them to the particular situation.[5]

In dealing with minor infractions the medical director may wish to consider a verbal reprimand, generally considered to be the least serious form of disciplinary action. If the verbal reprimand is applied properly, it can prevent a small problem from escalating into a major personnel problem. This type of action may or may not require documentation. At the medical director's discretion it may be documented using a memo, with one copy given to the individual and one copy kept by the medical director. This can be used as supporting evidence if problems continue to occur with the individual.

The formal written reprimand is the next step in the progression of disciplinary action. It is used to document a repeat offense of a minor problem or a more serious situation when suspension, demotion, or dismissal is not appropriate. Imperative for inclusion in this document is a comprehensive explanation of the corrective action or performance improvement expected from this individual, which should be written as a clearly defined objective. Having read and understood the objectives, the individual should sign the document.

Actions Needed

Suspension, demotion, and dismissal compose the subsequent steps in the disciplinary process. Although they still may be corrective, they are used as primary punitive measures for numerous repeated incidents or a single major one. It is the responsibility of the individual's supervisor and the medical director to stabilize the situation as rapidly as possible. This may include relieving the individual with pay until a decision is made concerning official action.

Essential to the process is not to commit to a particular form of disciplinary action prematurely. To ensure consistency of serious discipline administered throughout the organization, the department or agency director or chief should make the final decisions regarding suspension, demotion, or dismissal. Once again, the disciplinary process may be subject to civil service or legal action.

Alternatives

In some systems, medical directors are given the freedom to determine what action, if any, relative to the individual's certificate(s) should be taken as a result of the findings of the investigation.[4] The physician may place the individual on probation, suspend the individual's certificate to practice prehospital emergency care, or revoke or deny renewal of the individual's certificate.

The medical director for Orange County, Florida, may suspend a Prehospital Emergency Care Certificate if an infraction or performance deficiency indicates a need to temporarily remove the individual from the prehospital-care environment.[4] To protect the public health and safety the physician may suspend the certificate for a specified length of time until conditions for reinstatement are met. The Orange County medical director may also revoke or deny the renewal of a certificate if he determines that a deficiency is such that the individual should not be allowed to practice.

Similar disciplinary procedures are taken in Montgomery County, Md. The deciding body in the system may impose one or a combination of the following corrective actions:

1. Reclassification of paramedic status, including classification to internship or termination of paramedic status
2. Temporary suspension of paramedic duties, ranging from 30 days to 1 year
3. Recommendation to the State Board of Medical Directors for decertification of paramedic[3]

Medical directors are often given such latitude in the decision-making process since they often provide the authorization for an entire EMS system.

Summary

The function of a disciplinary policy is twofold: providing the timely and proper processing of disciplinary actions, and ensuring equity and fair treatment of employees in the issuing of such actions. A corrective, progressive, and lawful disciplinary policy is needed only when a link in the system has failed. It becomes the medical director's responsibility to guarantee consistent high-quality patient care while the providers conduct themselves in a highly self-disciplined manner.

REFERENCES

1. Davidson TD: Pre-hospital EMS lecture reference tables. Presented at the Quality Assurance in EMS Meeting, National Association of EMS Physicians, Clearwater, Fla, 1990.
2. Kenosha County Emergency Medical Services: *Disputes involving medical treatment,* In: *Kenosha County Emergency Medical Services Policies and Procedures,* 1990, The County.
3. Montgomery County, Maryland, Fire and Rescue Services: *Paramedic program standards,* In: *Emergency Medical Services,* 1981, The County.
4. Orange County EMSA: *Personnel: certification review process,* In: *Orange County EMSA policy procedure,* #460.00, March 1988, The County.
5. Phoenix Fire Department: *Employee discipline,* In: *Phoenix Fire Department administrative regulations,* MP 102.05, April 1990, The Department.
6. Prince George's County, Maryland, Fire Department: *Prince George's County (MD) Fire Department supervisor's guide to handling disciplinary matters,* 1990, The Department.

11

Funding Strategies for Quality Assurance Programs

Eric Davis, M.D.
Robert A. Swor, D.O.

Everybody agrees that quality assurance (QA) is necessary and desirable. Philip Crosby,[1a] in a book entitled *Quality is Free,* states:

> Quality has much in common with sex. Everybody is for it (under certain conditions, of course). Everyone feels they understand it (even though they wouldn't want to explain it). Everyone thinks execution is only a matter of following natural inclinations. And of course, most people feel that all problems in these areas are caused by other people.

One can probably add to this sentiment that no one feels the need to provide adequate funding for the program. This chapter discusses how a good quality improvement (QI) program is cost effective and suggests ways to help fund it.

Benefits of High Quality

The first step in a QA or QI program is to convince people of the need to ensure quality within the system. In business the cost of doing poor quality work is generally estimated to be between 12% and 20% of the cost of production. Major industrial leaders, such as Xerox, the Cadillac division of General Motors, and Federal Express, have made multimillion dollar commitments to quality in all operations because in the long run it is cost efficient and increases the ability to be competitive in the marketplace.

An example of how a good QI program can ultimately save money is International Telephone and Telegraph (ITT). In 1965 the company commissioned a study to examine the costs of each of the many components of its business. It discovered that a full 20% of the company's budget was spent on areas such as repairing and replacing defective equipment and performing inspections.

Following this rather startling discovery, ITT instituted a QI program. Although it started slowly and required an intense initial effort, the idea soon caught on and was embraced by the entire company. To check the effectiveness of QI on reducing costs, a follow-up study was commissioned in 1976. This time it was determined that only 2.5% of the budget was allocated to the tasks of repairing and replacing defective equipment and performing inspections— including the cost of the QI program. This resulted in an overall company savings of $530 million.[1a]

This same approach applies to the service industry. The Sheraton Hotel chain was reviewed by American Express and found to be one of the worst in terms of quality. This perception by clients was costing Sheraton a large portion of essential return business. Sheraton also undertook a QI program by educating and involving its employees, stressing the need of doing every aspect of the job correctly every time. Five years later Sheraton was rated as one of the best in quality, and its repeat (and therefore overall) business had increased dramatically.[1a]

The implications of this trend for emergency medical services (EMS) are clear: if quality medical care is rendered and efficient operations are developed, less time and money are spent in areas such as reeducation, risk management, materials management, absenteeism, and burnout. The system must be designed properly and continually refined, with the emphasis on improvement. As Crosby[1a] also states, "If the service is constructed and informed correctly, it follows that the operations of that company should be successful."

The data collected through a good QA system can also be used to determine sources of inefficiency. If unit-hour costs are high when compared with industry standards, the sources of inefficiency must be discovered so that improvement can occur.

One common area of excessive cost is staffing and scheduling patterns that do not take into account demand for service. Factors such as pattern fluctuations, inappropriate geographic deployment, poor redeployment procedures, and inefficient dispatch must be evaluated. Many of the new technologies currently available, such as computer-aided dispatch, vehicle tracking, and enhanced 9-1-1, should be considered and may reduce costs. In a two-tiered system these data can be used to monitor the appropriateness of decisions concerning the level of care that is provided to individual patients.

Another area of critical importance is preemployment screening. By identifying problems before hiring, the volume of employee turnover and the resultant increased costs can be minimized. Ambulance driving training and other injury prevention programs also result in savings in accidents averted, days lost to injury, and insurance premiums. An aggressive program implemented in Pinellas County, Fla., resulted in a 62% decrease in workmen's compensation claims and a 96% decrease in ambulance accidents.[8] The savings in these areas more than pay for the cost of the QI program. As funding decreases for EMS and all of health care, the need for greater efficiency of performance continues to grow.

The best measure of a successful EMS system is the level of care provided to the patient. That this care can and does improve patient outcome was recently demonstrated by Wuerz and Meador[15] in an abstract that showed improved short- and long-term outcome (defined as inpatient hospital stay) in patients receiving appropriate advanced life support prehospital care for congestive heart failure. The effectiveness of the medical director in improving patient outcome has also been demonstrated. Pepe,[6] in a Houston study conducted from 1983 to 1988, demonstrated improved survival rates from cardiac arrest after the addition of a full-time medical director. The positive effect of a QA plan was further borne out by a decrease in the number of patient care errors that resulted following the implementation of a systemwide QA plan.[11,13] Finally, errors in judgment by prehospital-care providers can be prevented through the involvement of online medical command, with the avoidance of potentially disastrous results.[16]

Aside from patient care issues, many health-care industry leaders have argued that QA is good risk management. Holroyd et al[5] argue in a landmark article that "the best defense against legal action is to design an EMS system that ensures medical accountability through complete offline and online medical direction."

History of EMS Funding

In the early days of EMS, funding was provided primarily through the government. Following the publication of the paper "Accidental Death & Disability: The Neglected Disease of Modern Society," federal funding for prehospital care became a priority.[2] The Highway Safety Act of 1966[1] provided initial funding through matching grant provisions to the states and provided for special demonstration projects. It thus served as a catalyst for the initiation of EMS systems and the development of public support and approval. The problem was that, except in a few instances, the program did not foster the development of *organized* EMS systems.

As knowledge about emergency care increased, it became apparent that patients would benefit from a regional approach to emergency care. Toward this end, in 1972 Congress approved funding for EMS demonstration projects in five regions to demonstrate how comprehensive EMS services could be supplied throughout a region. From 1972 to 1977 the Robert Wood Johnson Foundation funded projects on EMS response systems using well-defined access points (9-1-1) in 33 regions. A myriad of other federal projects (61 by one count) also existed during this period and were used for such purposes as training, disaster preparedness, communication systems, etc.[14]

The first comprehensive federal approach to supporting regional development of EMS systems came with the Emergency Medical Service Systems Act of 1973.[1] This act delineated the 15 mandatory components necessary in an EMS system and served as a template for program planners. It was designed to promote the development of systems that could "meet the individual characteristics of each community."

A total of $185 million was provided for 3 years and distributed to 303 regional lead agencies for disbursement. (The life of this act was prolonged until 1981 by amendments.) Each of these regions was to have a population of 700,000. The amount expected to be needed by each lead agency to develop a successful and a viable program was expected to be between $1.5 and $1.75 million (fiscal year 1974). Emphasis was placed on developing financial stability and securing alternative funding sources so that services would continue after federal funding ceased. Grants were disbursed as 1200 series grants for feasibility studies, initial operations, and evaluation and research. When funding for evaluation and research ceased, so did many evaluations of EMS care.[14]

This funding was dramatically reduced with the introduction of the Federal Block Grant programs in 1981. With this legislation, EMS funding was forced to compete for its share of the "block" funds with programs such as hypertension control, rodent control, rape prevention, crisis intervention, fluoridation, home health services, and health education. The manner in which these funds were distributed was left to the discretion of state authorities. The purpose of this legislation was to shift the responsibility of funding EMS services to the states, while still funding the lead agencies responsible for directing these services.

The outcome was a significant decrease in total EMS funding from 1981 to 1983. With this decrease, it became obvious that one of the chief failures of the EMS Act of 1973 was its inability to adequately stimulate local initiatives to fund EMS. As a result, many programs failed. Although funding rebounded through the mid-1980s, it is still up to EMS communities to compete with other constituencies for monies, and if EMS is not considered a high priority, funding suffers significantly.

General Funding Strategies

There are several general methods by which EMS systems are funded, which can in some cases provide specified monies for the QA process. The first method is federal support. Although federal monies for EMS systems have decreased, most states still receive significant funding. One survey reported that 35 states receive Public Health and Human Services (PHHS) funds for the provision of different aspects of EMS; 25 states receive funding through Department of Transportation Highway Safety Funds. In most cases these monies are provided through Section 402 of the Highway Safety Act for training of EMS personnel. In keeping with the intent of the PHHS act, funds are disbursed to lead agencies, which may use them for the statewide administration of EMS or for distribution to local agencies.[14]

Government Funding

State funding for EMS has become essential for the survival of many systems. Funding increased 50% from 1981 to 1985, according to a 1985 survey conducted by the Government Accounting Office.[7]

The methods involved in this funding vary greatly from state to state. Many states allocate monies from a general fund. Others, however, depend on various unique and creative methods. Dedicated EMS funds are provided by surcharges attached to motor vehicle registration, moving violations, driving-while-intoxicated violations, cigarettes, and other assessments (see Table 11-1). These funds may be used at the state level or may be redistributed to the local agencies. Additionally, the funds may be redistributed based on special needs, as with areas impacted by high tourism. This level of funding by the states is extremely variable, ranging from 3 cents per person in California to $1.20 in Alaska.[10]

One state that has a truly unique system is Maryland. Since its creation by executive order from the governor in 1973, the state funds the entire EMS system and provides for training (EMS personnel, nurses, and physicians), a statewide aeromedical transport system, tertiary care centers (most notably trauma), research, and statewide 9-1-1. This system receives its funding through the general fund and has recently added a surcharge on motor vehicle licenses to raise money for helicopter replacement.

Local funding is another universally important source of EMS revenue, and it is dependent on the local environment. Municipal systems generally tend to be supported by tax-generated revenue through the general fund, with these funds being augmented through service billings. Some regions provide EMS funds

Table 11-1. State Methods of EMS Funding

State	Method
Virginia Minnesota Idaho New Mexico	Revenue from vehicle or driver licensing
	Revenue from motor vehicle violations:
Florida	$5 per violation; $25 for driving while intoxicated
Arizona	$2.3 million/year from driving-while-intoxicated fines and other moving violations
Rhode Island	$1 surcharge per violation
Utah	$3 fee on fines or bail forfeiture
Mississippi	$5 fee per violation
Alabama	Cigarette taxes
Many states	Certification fees for EMTs and paramedics

through special assessments. Washington's King County, for example, voted a special tax millage to fund local EMS.

Subscription Services

Subscription service is another option. This works by offering the population the option of paying an annual fee, ranging from $2 to $60. Those who elect to subscribe receive EMS service without charge for the period covered by the subscription. Those without a subscription are charged on a fee-for-service basis.

In theory, subscription-based fees fund the deficit cost of the service (i.e., costs not covered by general revenues, insurance plans). One feature of the subscription plan is that it allows the provider to bill third-party payors for services rendered. The amount of the subscription fee is then determined by dividing the deficit projected by the number of subscriptions projected. An individual area may only expect a maximum subscription rate of 50% of the area's households (estimated by dividing the population served by 3), with the average being closer to 35% to 40%. Interestingly, the amount of the fee does not seem to affect the number of subscriptions except at the high and low extremes.[4]

Foundations

A similar approach to subscriptions is to solicit donations. This may only be done if the EMS service is a nonprofit organization, and it is commonly accomplished on the same form as is sent out for the subscription. Fundraising through donations has traditionally been the purview of small service organizations, which have raised funds for specific tangible projects, such as automatic defibrillator purchase and training. Foundations and local businesses may also be solicited for larger contributions, but these sources are often difficult to enlist because they are in high demand.

Some systems, such as the ones in San Francisco and Burbank, California, and in Everett, Washington, have had great success with separate foundations for EMS training and evaluation. Such foundations serve to tie a function easily supported by the community (e.g., training) with functions that are traditionally poorly funded (e.g., QA and research). Charitable gifts, grants, and bequests are often sources of revenue for these foundations. Fundraising for community-based programs, such as CPR training, has been very effective.

Third-Party Reimbursement

Third-party billing is also commonly used to generate EMS funds. The amount and the percentage of money supplied through this source are highly variable; Detroit generates only 20% of its budget in this manner, whereas Orange County, California, obtains 70% to 80% of its funding through direct billing.[3] EMS QA may not be directly billed in this manner, however, as it is specifically not covered in the Medicare Carriers Manual.[4] Instead, a specific CPT code exists for medical control, and some carriers reimburse for it. This only refers specifically to online medical direction of care for an individual patient. A service may, however, build a QA fee into its base rate by estimating the total cost of the QA process, then dividing this figure by the number of calls and adding it to the base rate. Systems should explore mechanisms to include QA fees into the costs of operations as a necessary item in the business of providing EMS care.

Public Utility Models

One of the most innovative approaches to funding medical control activities, including QA, is that employed by the public utility systems founded by Jack Stout.[12] These systems charge a set fee ($2 to $4) per patient transport for medical control functions. The systems are innovative in a number of respects. One unique provision is the restriction of service to one provider for both emergency and nonemergency transport within that region. Nonemergency transports serve to supplement the typically unprofitable emergency portion of EMS traffic. The public utility systems have been successful in a number of large regions, such as Tulsa, Oklahoma; Pinellas Co., Florida; Reno, Nevada; and Fort Wayne, Indiana.

Other Sources

Grants are another popular source of EMS funding. This constitutes "soft" money, in that grant money cannot be counted on as a dependable source of income and therefore should not be viewed as a source of continuing funding. Grants are an excellent source of seed money to start and to establish a program, particularly for some specific facet of the EMS system, such as QA.

A good way to view EMS funding is to use an organized approach to budgeting. The first step is to calculate direct income from such sources as federal and state funds, local taxes and subsidies, and reimbursed billing income. Direct income is stable and should not vary to a large degree. Once this is calculated, compare the figure to the estimated cost of providing EMS. The remaining deficit may be made up through subscriptions, donations, etc., with grants providing money for special projects. If the deficit is large, or if the deficit sources of funding are diminishing, then alternate ways of providing income, such as subsidies on motor vehicle violations, may be explored through the appropriate channels. The success of this process can be greatly enhanced if the positive effect of the EMS system can be demonstrated to the public. This is an important priority for a good QA program.

Summary

QA is an integral part of any EMS system, one that is particularly cost effective. The QA process documents the importance of EMS in the community, which may be crucial to obtaining funds from state and local governments, foundations, or even the population itself through subscription fees and donations. The program also serves to address concerns regarding existence of accountability and protection of the public against adverse outcomes.

Although the value of a QA plan—and the money it saves—is apparent only after the system is functioning properly, there are many varied and creative methods to help pay for the QA program on an ongoing basis. Once the value of the QA plan becomes apparent, systems will not wonder how they can pay for QA, but instead how they cannot.

REFERENCES

1. Boyd DR: *The history of emergency medical systems in the United States of America.* In Boyd DR, Edlich RF, Micks N, editors: *Systems approach to emergency medical care,* 1983, Appleton-Century-Crofts.
1a. Crosby P: *Quality is free: the art of making quality certain,* New York, 1979, McGraw-Hill.
2. Division of Medical Services: *Accidental death and disability: the neglected division of modern society,* National Academy of Sciences—National Research Council, 1966, Washington, D.C.
3. Drake L, Thompson M: *Systems design and human resources in prehospital care.* In Cleary V, Wilson R, editors: *Administrative and clinical management,* Rockville, Md, 1987, Aspen Publishers.
4. Henry JR: *Practical alternative for providers of pre-hospital care: ambulance service,* Management seminar handout, Ross Westview Emergency Medical Services Authority, Ross Township, Pa, 1990.
5. Holyroyd B, Knopp R, Kallsen G: Medical control: quality assurance in prehospital care, *JAMA* 256:1027-31, 1986.
6. Pepe P et al: The impact of intense physician supervision on the effectiveness of an emergency medical services system, *Ann Emerg Med* 17(7):752, 1988 (abstract).
7. Report assesses leadership of states in providing EMS, *EMS Communicator* 13(6):1-4, 1986.
8. Schrader D: *Funding the program.* Presented at National Association of EMS Physicians Winter Meeting, Clearwater, Fla, January 1991.
9. Smith J: Financial considerations in emergency medical services systems, *Emerg Med Clin North Am* 8(1):155-63, 1990.
10. State and province survey, *Emerg Med Serv* 19(12):221-251, 1990.
11. Stewart RD et al: A computerized quality assurance system for an emergency medical service, *Ann Emerg Med* 14:25-29, 1985.
12. Stout J: System financing in principles of EMS systems. In Rousch W, editor: *A comprehensive test for physicians,* Dallas, 1989, American College of Emergency Physicians.
13. Swor R, Hoelzer M: A computer-assisted quality assurance audit in a multiprovider EMS system, *Ann Emerg Med* 19(3):286-290, 1990.
14. Swor R: Funding strategies for EMS systems. In Kuehl AE, editor: *NAEMSP EMS medical directors handbook,* St. Louis, 1989, Mosby-Year Book.
15. Wuerz R, Meador S: Effect of prehospital medications on mortality and length of stay, *Ann Emerg Med* 20(4):447, 1991 (abstract).
16. Zehner W et al: Non-transport of prehospital patients: is stronger medical control needed? *Ann Emerg Med* 20(4):446, 1991 (abstract).

Section Three

Quality Assessment in Different Environments

Efforts to improve quality have been undertaken in every type of EMS system and in a variety of environments. The authors in this section describe quality assurance efforts in each of their respective systems, with discussion of the needs and limitations of each environment. Ideas are presented for special consideration in program development, and methods are suggested as currently used. Because the solutions to issues raised are as unique as individual EMS systems, "cookbook" problem-solving approaches are not given. Methods used in trauma systems and air medical services are presented so that they can be integrated into the entire EMS system's quality efforts.

12

Quality Assurance for Urban EMS

Vincent Mosesso, M.D.

Developing and implementing a comprehensive program of quality assurance (QA) in an urban emergency medical services (EMS) system involves a number of unique challenges. The size and complexity of such systems mandate that the medical director and the others charged with this task gain insight into a variety of important factors. He must understand the system's administration, personnel, finances, geography, and demography, as well as its niche in the local political structure. The urban venue presents difficulties in procuring the commitment and the authority necessary for an effective quality improvement (QI) program. The large call volume and the number of personnel require sophisticated methods of data management, which can be greatly enhanced through computerization. The final but most important challenge is to use the information gained through the QA process to make real and meaningful improvements in the system's delivery of patient care. This chapter elaborates on these various elements as they apply to the urban setting.

Special Characteristics Influencing Quality Assurance in Urban EMS

To discuss QA in urban EMS one must first define the term "urban." Although an intuitive sense of which areas fit this designation may be common, finding an exact definition is difficult. According to one source:

> The city may be regarded as a relatively permanent concentration of population, together with its diverse habitations, social arrangements, and supporting activities, occupying a more or less discrete site, and having a cultural importance that differentiates it from other types of human settlement and association.[5]

Thus every urban environment is a unique synthesis of many sociologic factors. Comprehension of these factors is necessary to develop an efficient, effective QI plan for the local urban EMS system.

Environment

Perhaps the single characteristic that most clearly separates urban from suburban and rural is population *density*, as there are suburban systems that serve populations larger than some cities. A significant subset of that population is indigent and uneducated, and lives in overcrowded conditions. The clustering of non-English speaking immigrants as well as the occurrence of increased drug trafficking and associated violence also present special challenges and hazards.

Another urban phenomenon that challenges the urban EMS system is the marked fluctuation in the service area's population as a result of the daily influx of suburban-dwelling commuters. Shifts also occur between the downtown and the residential neighborhoods within the city. These fluxes in total population and density necessitate adaptive patterns of unit staffing and deployment.

Providers with the urban EMS system encounter a distinctive physical environment. A clustering of high-rise structures, business establishments, and congested, narrow streets comprise a central hub that presents a variety of difficulties for system response and patient access and transfer. Other areas of the city may house industrial complexes that offer mechanical, electrical, or chemical hazards. There are often a large number of heavily traveled express-ways, some with limited access points. Still other neighborhoods may be densely packed residential areas with both single- and multiple-family dwellings.

Proper response to such scenes necessitates special preparation. An index of pertinent building layouts (including such things as location of stairwells, ventilation ducts, and fire suppression hoses), elevator access codes, and other relevant information should be on board every response unit. Current street maps and daily traffic reports reduce unnecessary response delays; good relations with the police department are also helpful in this regard. Provision of protective gear, such as bulletproof vests, must be considered, as should safety and self-defense training. Each system must evaluate the special needs presented by its particular service area. In Pittsburgh, for example, a tragic drowning led to the establishment of a water rescue team comprised of EMS, fire, and police personnel.

Special events are also common in the urban setting; the EMS system is frequently faced with mass gatherings that necessitate a great deal of advance planning and resource procurement. A dramatic example of the efficacy of such planning was the successful response to a boating accident during a Pittsburgh regatta.[28]

Personnel and Medical Leadership

Urban systems generally consist of a large number of field personnel, which creates difficulties from a QA perspective. The capacity of the medical director to observe individual paramedics and to maintain significant personal contact is tremendously jeopardized. Fortunately, in most urban areas there is an adequate number of interested and qualified physicians to assist the director in this role. Although more supervisory and administrative personnel are also usually available, direct involvement by physicians is essential.[16]

A mechanism should be developed to allow for timely and noncumbersome communications between the urban EMS field personnel and the medical director. This could include direct mailings between the two parties, scheduled office time for telephone calls and office appointments, occasional field visits to medic stations, and open forums or lunches with the director. Stewart[24] noted that "the role of the physician in EMS must include a consistent, visible, in-the-street presence that almost always will result in widespread acceptance by field teams, greater support for medical policies, and more rigid adherence by field teams to prehospital protocols." Yet even when all these efforts are made, there is still the risk that individual medics will feel dissociated from the medical director, thereby eroding the director's ability to maintain tight medical control.

Urban systems are either governmental agencies or agencies contracted by government. Because both employ full-time personnel, this offers certain advantages in the QA process. One can establish requirements and then recruit and select personnel who best fit the needs and the operational structure of the particular system.[4] Initial training and continuing education should be easier to arrange than in systems comprised mostly of volunteers or part-time personnel, provided that adequate finances are available. Also, urban medics typically handle more calls per shift and perform more skilled procedures than their suburban or rural counterparts. Thus individual medic profiles of skill performance, ECG interpretation, protocol deviations, and similar parameters can be more rapidly developed.

Additionally, because of the power inherent in the employer-employee relationship, greater control and discipline can be exerted by a system with full-time paid personnel. However, the degree to which the medical director shares in this power may vary as a result of political and financial relationships, as well as contractual provisions. Although the medical director clearly should not be involved in discipline concerning nonmedical system policies and procedures, the ability to exercise some meaningful form of discipline with regard to medical care issues is appropriate and, indeed, necessary.

Unionism

Another issue that complicates directing and interacting with large groups of full-time personnel is unionism. Although unions certainly have legitimate roles and functions, they can also create difficulties when implementing a QA program. An obvious example would be an overly defensive posture that antagonizes attempts at personnel evaluation and corrective action. An indirect limitation may result from preexisting clauses in the union contract restricting or limiting the ability to implement certain changes that may be clearly beneficial from a medical viewpoint. Examples of such would be strictly defined, inflexible job descriptions and language that inhibits or prevents changing structural system components, often in an attempt to preserve specific positions. Indeed, the medical director may find himself "caught" between the union and the political or the administrative leadership of the EMS system.

A biting example of such an unfortunate situation was experienced during the Pittsburgh EMS strike of 1986. Although the medical director was a strong advocate of the field paramedics and certainly agreed with the union position that they were greatly underpaid, he was also responsible for the provision of quality prehospital care to the 450,000 area residents and approximately 1 million daily visitors to the city. Thus the medical director's legal and ethical duties to his paramedic colleagues were in direct conflict with his duties to the city's residents. A new medical director would do well to learn the history and the current perspective of the EMS union or unions in his locale; certainly every effort should be made to maintain open communication with the union leadership.

Financial and Political

Other factors that impinge on QA activities are the urban political and financial settings. Although a full discussion of these aspects is beyond the scope of this text, the key concept is that QA must be regarded as an integral component of the system and must receive adequate budgetary support (i.e., a designated line item). The medical director must clearly and emphatically support this principle. In the face of a shrinking tax base as a result of the continued flight to the suburbs and the decreased federal support for cities, QA is often seen as an easy target by administrators. There must be a commitment from both the medical director and the administrative chief to expend the necessary time, effort, and funds. It is also critically important that the director have the authority to implement a comprehensive plan and to enact changes based on findings of the QA process.[21] The QA program must be treated as necessary for facilitating evaluation and change in the system and assuring accountability to the populace it serves.

In contrast to suburban systems that use staff physicians from local emergency departments, urban EMS systems often contract with or employ a full-time medical director. Although compensation may allow for greater commitment (especially in terms of time), the political and the monetary ties that this creates can place the medical director in a compromising position. The medical director should be free to take positions and to implement changes based on patient care issues, although the realities of political and fiscal limitations must be appreciated. Political savvy and an ability to interact artfully with important government, administrative, and community leaders are prerequisites.

Research

Although research can be undertaken in any size or type of EMS system, the greater call volume and the frequent association with university hospitals and residency training programs typically lead to more active research in urban systems. Research activities yield positive benefits beyond the direct results of the studies themselves; these benefits include better physician involvement, heightened awareness and greater depth of knowledge of the problem being studied, and often a boost in morale as field personnel are involved in state-of-the-art and pioneering practices. It also serves as the catalyst for change, not only for the system being studied, but also for the field of EMS. Most changes in the practice of EMS in this country are a direct result of urban EMS research. Research should be considered a legitimate component of the QI program.

Media

Urban EMS systems are frequently placed in the spotlight of the local and the national media, more so than in suburban communities. Although media exposure and relations do not directly impact on the quality of care rendered by the system, issues such as response time, individual case management, and overall system management may be aired publicly. This scrutiny demands that an internal mechanism exists to ensure quality.

Although the QA program must function independent of media pressure, congenial relations with the press reduce external interference, which can disrupt the operation of the system. Close surveillance by the media also necessitates that special efforts be made to maintain confidentiality, not only of QA activities but also of systemwide operations. All personnel should be advised upfront of the system's policy regarding interaction with the media.

Special Problems in Urban EMS

System Abuse

Another problem found primarily in large and midsized urban systems is overutilization or "system abuse." Braun[1] reported that the average nontransport rate among 20 midsized urban systems is 38%, whereas Luterman[13] reported that paramedics actually rendered treatment in only 20% of their responses. This is due in part to the large indigent population possessing limited awareness of and access to other sources of primary health care. Nevertheless, improper use of EMS resources is clearly deleterious. Such calls not only waste resources but also place unnecessary stress on both the personnel and the system itself; they severely hamper efforts at maintaining morale.

Thus system abuse must be addressed as a quality-of-care issue. Many systems have tolerated overuse as a result of the potential legal exposure from call-screening programs, as exemplified by a well-publicized event in which a nurse who was screening refused to send an ambulance to an initial call for help, after which the patient died.[2] However, the development of sophisticated "priority dispatch" systems involving special training of dispatchers allows for disciplined and defendable use of resources.[2,3,10]

Nontransport calls are clearly potential legal and patient care land mines requiring both prospective and retrospective attention.[6] At least one system has found it necessary to require online command for all nontransports.[29] Field personnel assessments and their resultant documentation must clearly reflect the patient's competency status, as well as detailed history and physical exam findings, including vital signs.[12,22] Trip reports concerning nontransported patients should be just as complete, if not more so, than reports for transported patients.

Hospital Destination

Urban systems enjoy the advantage of having multiple emergency departments and specialty centers within their service area. Transport times are usually short, and the need to decide between ground transport to a local emergency department or to a more distant specialty center or helicopter evacuation is obviated. However, the multiplicity of hospitals with varying levels of specialty expertise requires that destination policies be set prospectively for field personnel. These guidelines must be formulated carefully with input from affected hospitals. The process should also involve the directors of area emergency departments and specialty services, such as trauma, burns, complicated obstetrics, and neonatal resuscitation. Some emergency departments strongly prefer not to receive certain cases (e.g., pregnant trauma patients), deferring to nearby centers better equipped and staffed to care for such patients.

As demand for specialty services and emergency services as a whole increases, the ability for a specific hospital to supply those services has at times become overwhelmed. Institutions in many cities, especially large metropolitan areas, have experienced tremendous problems with emergency department over-crowding. This has affected and continues to affect the ability of these hospitals to accept and to manage EMS patients. Most systems have developed methods of diverting ambulances from an otherwise appropriate destination. Although this practice has not been studied extensively, it appears to be safe.[30] Protocols must be developed to ensure that ambulance diversion is performed only in instances in which patient care is not compromised. A system must also be developed to monitor this process.

In summary, the QA process must ensure the appropriateness of patient destinations; this involves prospectively establishing destination and diversion policies and retrospectively reviewing their implementation and effectiveness.

Developing Specific Components of Urban Quality Assurance

It is especially important in urban EMS systems with complex administrative structures and a large number of personnel that representatives from *every* level of the system become involved in the QA task. The Deming model[11] holds that it is vital to include field personnel in the process. For example, the recently formed QA committee in the Pittsburgh EMS system is comprised of this author and another faculty physician as co-chair, seven rank-and-file field medics, two training division medics, and a supervisor representing administration. Committee meetings are open to all field personnel. This broad-based involvement facilitates identification of important issues, cultivates acceptance of QA findings, and serves as an important source of information regarding specific field information. It is also crucial in setting priorities from the standpoint of improving patient care. A summary of an urban EMS system QA plan is presented in Table 12-1.

System Structure

Urban EMS systems currently exist in a variety of organizational structures; most are combined with the fire service, some are third services, and some cities contract with a private firm. Response structure may be one- or two-tiered, and advanced life support (ALS) providers may or may not respond in transport units. Call volume per unit may vary dramatically from 0.9 to 5.2 calls/10,000 population/day.[1] The important concept is that the structure should allow for the most efficient use of personnel and vehicles—the exact formulation depends on local geographic, demographic, and financial conditions.

The QA program must track response times, not just the mean time but also the percent of calls answered within a designated time standard. Response times to ALS calls and the percent availability of an ALS unit for ALS-required calls should be tracked. This issue is of particular importance in urban systems as a result of the high call volume and the temporal as well as the geographic population fluxes that were discussed earlier in this chapter.[14] With the evolving importance of automated defibrillation, response times for first-responder units must also be tracked. Although EMS systems traditionally track only their own times, attention must be paid to important adjuvant personnel. Prompt response of police and rescue squads is essential for the safety and the effective functioning of EMS personnel.

Dispatch

Perhaps the most important factor affecting operating efficiency is dispatch. One advantage of urban systems is that a single central dispatch center coordinates a large fleet of units, allowing for more efficient systems management. Urban dispatch centers generally handle a much higher call volume than their suburban counterparts. The high level of efficiency required can be achieved through the use of modern computerized systems.

Because urban systems in particular are burdened with such a large percentage of low-urgency calls, interest is rising in prioritized dispatch programs that are believed to allow for more appropriate use of resources.[3,10] Many systems are providing prearrival instructions as well.

Table 12-1. Urban EMS QA Plan

Component	Prospective	Concurrent	Retrospective
Structure	Usually preexisting Determine service area needs Procure appropriate vehicles/supplies Determine best deployment Establish communications system Ensure appropriate support and backup (such as fire, rescue, police) available	On-duty supervisor ensures best use of resources	Analyze: • response times (including for specific areas and times of day) • availability of advanced life support when needed • calls/unit/shift
Dispatch	Determine need for computer-aided dispatch and priority dispatch Develop emergency medical dispatch system and train dispatchers	"Flip cards" to guide dispatchers Supervisor at dispatch center monitors calls pending and prioritizes	Track pertinent time intervals: • call placed until answered • answered until dispatched Track proper priority designation
Personnel (including first responders)	Establish preemployment and employment requirements Provide appropriate specialized training needs, based on demands on system	Supervisor or physician on scene or by radio report	Review of specific calls Develop "Medic Profile": Procedures, cases seen, continuing education Determine specific continuing education needs Computerized data base essential

Continued

Component	Prospective	Concurrent	Retrospective
Patient care (systems issues)	Ensure proper training Develop protocols and update regularly Establish/review list of approved meds/Rx's Establish destination guidelines for specialty cases	Supervisor or physician on scene or by radio report	Review sampling of calls Focused review on specific types of calls, such as chest pain or cardiac arrest, on regular basis Track overall events and frequency of procedures and success rates Track protocol violations Track time to defibrillate and other critical times
Medical command	Train command physicians Familiarize physicians with protocols and available drugs/equipment Introduce physicians to medics	Medical director monitors sampling Residents/new command physicians monitored by faculty/experienced physicians	Review command sheets—focus on protocol deviations, appropriateness of orders Base station audits
Medical control	Set up agreement outlining duties, responsibilities, and authority base (ensure independence) Choose physician with predetermined qualifications	Chief must involve medical director in all system decisions that impact on delivery of care	Regular review of medical direction activities by quality assurance committee

The QA program must closely evaluate dispatch operations, specifically by tracking time intervals (receipt by call taker to transfer to dispatcher, receipt by dispatcher to notification of response units, and unit notification to arrival at scene), reviewing the appropriateness of priority designations, and ensuring the appropriate use of system resources. Pittsburgh paramedics assign a priority level (e.g., life-threatening, urgent, or nonurgent) *after* each call; the paramedic's designation is then compared to the level assigned by the call taker *before* dispatch. It should be noted that retrospectively and prospectively assigned designations may differ but both be correct. An EMS supervisor onsite at the emergency operations center has been shown to be an effective concurrent control as well.

Protocols and Equipment

Good QA requires prospective development of protocols and specification of equipment, supplies, and medications. These protocols and equipment requirements should reflect the short transport times in urban settings and include guidelines that designate appropriate hospital destinations for specialty cases (as discussed earlier). As an example, ongoing research may find that prehospital use of thrombolytic therapy for acute myocardial infarction is indicated in rural or suburban systems but not in urban systems. Similarly, data regarding medication use may indicate that use of some drugs is infrequent and does or does not justify their availability in the EMS system.

The higher volume of calls per medic in most urban systems may influence which procedures medics are permitted to perform and how far along in the protocol they may proceed before contacting medical command. However, the rarity of true communication equipment failure would allow for a more stringent requirement to contact medical command.

Medical Command

Strong systemwide medical direction is the *sine qua non* for ensuring quality patient care. Nevertheless, the value of physician online command has been questioned, especially in busy systems with full-time field personnel. Indeed, several published reports have found that medical control infrequently alters paramedic protocols, and some authors have argued that contacting command unnecessarily prolongs scene time.[8,19] However, a recent retrospective review of the Kansas City, Missouri, system disputes this position.[7]

From a QA perspective, online command has many attractive features. The most important advantage is that it allows for *concurrent* medical control, albeit generally remote from the scene. Command physicians are able to immediately evaluate the individual paramedic's patient assessment and care plan, while still maintaining an overall sense of field operations (i.e., "what's going on out there"). Online command also provides for more frequent paramedic-physician interaction, which is vital but easily lost in urban systems.

An affiliation with emergency medicine training programs and the greater availability of physicians interested in EMS may allow for actual on-scene medical command and supervision. As an example, the Pittsburgh EMS system uses postgraduate year-II and postgraduate year-III emergency medicine residents to respond to patients with cardiac arrest, unstable cardiac arrhythmias, respiratory failure, vehicle entrapment, and multiple-casualty incidents.[23] This program of physician response is facilitated by a high volume of calls in a confined geographic area. Clearly, direct on-scene observation of paramedic activities is the ultimate QA tool.[16,24]

Of vital importance, although often neglected, is the assurance of quality medical command and medical direction. Some system should be in place to review orders and reports taken by online medical command. This task requires the personal involvement of the medical director. An excellent description of a base-station audit program has been published.[17] If residents are used in providing command, concurrent QA through the use of faculty supervisors is an excellent approach.

Finally, the medical director himself must be open to scrutiny; this may be accomplished by the use of a QA committee comprised of field paramedics and administrative personnel, as discussed earlier.

Personnel Evaluation

Because of the high volume of urban EMS calls, use of a computerized data base for creating individual medic profiles can be invaluable in tracking the number of calls, the types of cases, the attempted and the successfully performed procedures, the continuing education programs, and the other QA matters.[12] Supervisors should be used for moment-to-moment operations management, as well as on-scene observation of field personnel in lieu of physician response. Periodic sessions with the medical director and clinical time spent in pertinent hospital units (although often balked at by full-time medics) are valuable to both the medic and the supervising physicians.

A QA program must also evaluate the care provided by first responders. Although non-ALS personnel have traditionally not fallen under the medical director's umbrella, first-responder activities are clearly part of the care provided by the system and must fall under medical QA. This is particularly true for systems with automated defibrillation programs.

Data Collection

Although retrospective review is considered the weakest form of QA, it is easy to perform and it does yield valuable information. Given the volume of data from modern EMS systems, a modern, state-of-the-art QA program all but demands use of computers for expedient and accurate data collection and analysis (see Chapter 9). Several examples of such use of computers have been described in the literature.[25,26,27] Certain information, such as response time and nature of complaint, should be tabulated for every call, along with identifiers for pertinent case groupings. Optically scanned forms greatly increase the efficiency of this process, although such systems are prone to logistical problems.[9] Urban systems may also have the benefit of affiliation with universities and larger governmental agencies, which have greater data-handling capabilities.

At a minimum a system must exist to review a sampling of calls to ensure a reasonable standard of care and adequate documentation. Incidents and complaints must also be reviewed and are often valuable sources of information regarding system problems. In addition, specific types of cases may be retrieved for more intensive periodic review. Cases are usually selected because they occur at high frequency (such as nontransports), carry significant risk (such as respiratory failure or chest pain), or occur at low frequency but involve extremely high risk (such as complicated obstetrics). Periodic reviews may also be developed in response to recent developments (e.g., a rash of unrecognized esophageal intubations).

Summary

Urban EMS systems, although sharing much in common with their suburban and rural counterparts, are affected by a number of factors unique to the city environment. The size and complexity of urban systems present many challenges to organizing and maintaining an effective and efficient QA program, but they also enable these systems to provide the most efficient and advanced prehospital care possible.

REFERENCES

1. Braun O, McCallion R: Characteristics of midsized urban EMS systems, *Ann Emerg Med* 19(5):536-546, 1990.
2. Clawson J, Dernocoeur K: *Principles of emergency medical dispatch,* Englewood Cliffs, NJ, 1988, The Brady Co.
3. Curka PA et al: Computer-aided EMS priority dispatch: ability of a computerized triage system to safely spare paramedics from responses not requiring A.L.S., *Ann Emerg Med* 20(4):446, 1991.
4. Dick T: Quality assurance: an endless pursuit of excellence, *J Emerg Med Serv* (March) 32-36, 1988.
5. *Encyclopedia Britannica,* ed 15, vol. 16, Chicago, 1990.
6. Goldberg RJ et al: A review of prehospital care litigation in a large metropolitan EMS system, *Ann Emerg Med* 19(5):557-561, 1990.
7. Gratton ML et al: Effect of standing orders on paramedic scene time for trauma patients, *Ann Emerg Med* 20(12):1306-1309, 1991.
8. Hoffman JR, Luo JS, Schinger DL: Does paramedic hospital base radio contact result in actions that deviate from standard diagnosis protocols? *West J Med* 153:283-287, 1990.
9. Joyce SM, Brown DE: An optically scanned EMS reporting form and analysis system for stationwide use: development and 5 years experience, *Ann Emerg Med* 20(12):1325-1330, 1991.

10. Kallsen G, Nabors MD: The use of priority medical dispatch to distinguish between high and low risk patients, *Ann Emerg Med* 19(4):458-459, 1990.
11. Kritchevsky SB, Simmons BP: Continuous quality improvement, concepts and applications for physician care, *JAMA* 266(13):1817-1823, 1991.
12. Lavoie FW: Consent, involuntary treatment, and use of force in an urban emergency department, *Ann Emerg Med* 21(1):25-32, 1992.
13. Luterman A et al: Evaluation of prehospital emergency medical service (EMS): defining areas for improvement, *J Trauma* 23(8):702-708, 1983.
14. Mayer JD: EMS delays, response time and survival, *Med Care* 17(8):818-827, 1979.
15. Ornato JP et al: Impact of improved emergency medical services and emergency trauma care on the reduction in mortality from trauma, *J Trauma* 25(7):575-579, 1985.
16. Pepe PE, Stewart RD: Role of the physician in the prehospital setting, *Ann Emerg Med* 15(12):1480-1483, 1986.
17. Pointer JE: The ALS base hospital audit for medical control in an EMSS, *Ann Emerg Med* 16(5):557-560, 1987.
18. Pointer JE, Osor MA: EMS QA: a computerized incident reporting system, *J Emerg Med* 5:513-517, 1987.
19. Pointer JE, Osor M, Campbell C: The impact of standing orders on medication and skill selection, paramedic assessment, and hospital outcome, *Prehospital and Disaster Medicine* 6(3):303-308, 1991.
20. Polsky SS, Weigand JV: Quality assurance in emergency medical systems, *Emerg Med Clin North Am* 8(1):75-84, 1990.
21. Ryan J: *Quality assurance in emergency medical services systems.* In Kuehl AE, editor: *EMS medical directors handbook,* St. Louis, 1989, Mosby–Year Book.
22. Selden BS, Schnitzer PG, Nolan FX: Medicolegal documentation of prehospital transport, *Ann Emerg Med* 19(5):547-551, 1990.
23. Stewart RD: Design of a resident in-field experience for an emergency medicine residency curriculum, *Ann Emerg Med* 16(2):175-179, 1987.
24. Stewart RD: Medical direction in emergency medical services: the role of the physician, *Emerg Med Clin North Am* 5(1):119-132, 1987.
25. Stewart RD et al: A computer-assisted QA system for an EMS system, *Ann Emerg Med* 14(1):25-29, 1985.
26. Swor RA, Hoelzer M: A computer-assisted quality assurance audit in a multiprovider EMS system, *Ann Emerg Med* 19(3):286-290, 1990.
27. Valenzuela TD et al: Computer modeling of emergency medical system performance, *Ann Emerg Med* 19(8):898-901, 1990.
28. Vukmir RB, Paris PM: The Three Rivers regatta accident, an EMS Perspective, *Am J Emerg Med,* 9(1):64-71, 1991.
29. Zehner WJ et al: Non-transport of prehospital patients: is stronger medical control needed? *Ann Emerg Med,* 20(4):446, 1991.
30. Zydlo S: *Diversions and bypass.* In Kuehl AE, editor: *EMS medical directors handbook,* St. Louis, 1989, Mosby–Year Book.

13

EMS Quality Assurance in Rural Environments

Kathleen A. Cline, M.D.

Current EMS quality assurance (QA) literature regarding prehospital care is based largely on urban systems. These areas are typically served by a full-time, paid, professional paramedic service, with high call volume, sophisticated dispatch systems, short transport distances, and multiple receiving hospitals. The medical director may have an extensive supportive network for maintaining quality care, including computerized data collection, in-field auditors, and offline office staff.[14] In contrast, a rural medical director is less likely to have such resources,[15] and yet he remains responsible for a system that extends over a much greater area.

Clearly, rural systems are not equivalent to sprawling urban systems. Geographic factors are considerably different, as are the population profile, the types of emergencies, and the principles of field triage.[5,17] In areas such as eastern North Carolina, 15% to 30% of the population have incomes below the national poverty level.[7] System access remains a major problem in rural areas. From the time that the emergency occurs hours may pass before the victim is discovered and the passerby is able to gain access to a telephone. Many areas have neither 9-1-1 nor a centralized 7-digit emergency telephone number. The passerby may not be able to define his location; many locales are identified by local landmarks, and county routes are largely unnamed. Furthermore, residences exist that do not have addresses, and many people use post office boxes in town for their mail, making locating the caller difficult even with enhanced 9-1-1 service.[5,16] Response times may be prolonged further if the incident is some distance from a road, requiring the responders to carry equipment, medications, and radios by foot. One paramedic recalled a run in which the last mile was "on foot, through the swamp to this hunter who was having an MI [myocardial infarction]; we were up to our thighs in snakes and swamp, it was pitch dark, and we just prayed he wouldn't code." Is it reasonable to expect an 8-minute response time under such circumstances? Obviously, urban EMS system models are not applicable to this setting.

Rural emergencies have a different profile as well. In this author's area, many people do not seek medical care unless they are critically ill; it is not uncommon to see a 50-year-old person who has never seen a physician before arrive in pulmonary edema. Penetrating trauma occurs much less often in rural areas than in concentrated urban areas; a higher proportion of penetrating trauma is self-inflicted suicide attempts or accidental hunting injuries. On the other hand, vehicular trauma tends to be severe; a person involved in a rural motor vehicle crash is 3 times more likely to sustain serious injury than an urban crash victim.[2,16] (This may be due to poorer driving conditions and higher speed limits.) There is also a greater use of jeeps and pickup trucks, which are associated with higher death rates. Agricultural machinery injuries are more frequently seen in farming areas.[8]

Field triage and transport protocols must take into account the availability of regionalized specialty centers. In most rural settings there is no choice but to go to the nearest hospital, which typically is the only hospital in the area. Even then many facilities do not have in-house, 24-hour physician coverage.[16] Issues such as diversion and field triage become moot, except in areas where an advanced-level aeromedical team is available to respond quickly to a scene. Additional training in triage is necessary so that responding ground crews can quickly identify such a situation (usually trauma) and request dispatch of the aeromedical team, which may transport the victim directly to a more distant tertiary care center.

Rural Emergency Medical Response

In rural settings, and particularly in wilderness areas, ambulances are staffed primarily by basic emergency medical technicians (EMTs), even though, ironically, there is a much greater need for advanced prehospital service. In urban areas most technicians are paid, whereas in rural areas most volunteer. Without these volunteers, many communities would not be able to provide any EMS at all.[16] Volunteer EMTs are a diminishing resource, primarily because of the restraints of economics and time.[1] Yet they are a valuable resource—a decidedly dedicated group who spend most of their nonemployed time on some aspect of EMS. A community-based squad is a tightly knit group of neighbors who know each other well and share a sense of pride and singular purpose rarely seen in contemporary society.[3] Society has changed; few people are available to volunteer during weekdays, and people from rural communities may commute well out of their districts to their jobs. These factors have created a crisis in daytime EMS service. Squads are struggling to cover the daytime schedule, and many have reluctantly begun to use paid daytime help.[12,16] Resources for training and continuing education may not be locally available, creating further disincentive.[11,16]

Rural EMS Medical Directors

Most emergency medicine residency programs are based at large regional medical centers. Consequently, most potential EMS medical directors are trained within sophisticated, large EMS systems. It is little wonder then that a residency-trained, "hot-shot" doctor may not be well received in a rural volunteer basic EMS squad, which has gotten along just fine without a medical director. The principles learned in residency do not seem to apply in a rural area, and a physician may be somewhat bewildered at the less-than-embracing reception.

A medical director must establish credibility with the EMS community. Otherwise, attempts at implementing change may be ignored or met with passive (but powerful) resistance. In many rural cultures educational degrees are less important than dedication and hard work. This concept is reinforced daily, especially in a volunteer-based system. In return, the EMT is motivated by strong psychological factors, such as a sense of belonging to an important group, a sense of challenge, a sense of helping someone in need, and a sense of self-esteem that comes from recognition.[3,12,13] When the medical director is as dedicated as the EMT constituency, effective influence surfaces.

Does the medical director participate in routine field care in the field? Is he with the others in the ditch trying to get an IV started? Does the medical director participate in regular squad meetings, depriving his family of an evening at home with him as other staff members routinely do? These demonstrations of commitment are the keys to earning respect, acceptance, and authority. Furthermore, such participation is educational and may affect the medical director's concept of rural prehospital care. He may come to appreciate what really can and cannot be done in the field and understand better the differences between prehospital and emergency department medicine.

Ensuring Quality Medical Care in the Rural Environment

Traditionally, QA has been described in three parts: prospective, concurrent, and retrospective. Prospective QA involves written protocols, system policies, and EMT education. These should be clearly defined, measurable, and consistent. With rare exception, patient care should follow the protocols, and any deviations need to be carefully documented and reviewed. Protocols must include basic life support care to ensure consistency during the entire patient interaction. Volunteer squads have a high turnover rate for personnel.[12] This, coupled with a low call volume, results in a relatively small experience base for each provider. Explicit protocols leave little room for assumption and serve as an educational device for new squad members.

Concurrent QA implies assessing the delivery of care as it is being *delivered*. This is difficult in a low-volume, rural setting. It is impractical to "ride along" when the truck may not be dispatched for several hours or even days. The medical director, or designated field supervisor, may more typically co-respond to a dispatch heard on the scanner. This is an invaluable experience for the medical director in that it quickly identifies field problems and their source. For instance, when the patient arrives at the hospital without a cervical collar (which you thought was indicated), how would you know if this error was due to inadequate training, a personality conflict within the team, or an unusual scenario justifying the omission? Procedural technique can be best assessed this way as well. An alternative to being on site is to routinely audiotape all critical calls and then review the audio tapes. This is an excellent way to assess how the team functions as a whole, how long it took to intubate the patient, how organized the team was, how they interacted with the patient, and so on. It is also useful for identifying educational needs.[10] Tape recordings of the EMTs' radio report to the hospital can also be useful.

Finally, retrospective QA can assist in analyzing protocol deviations and devising areas for continuing education. It is of limited effectiveness in truly assessing the adequacy of the care delivered. More often it simply assesses the adequacy of documentation.

A common trap into which medical directors can fall lies in believing that the standards of care must be low because "they are volunteers, and if criticized, they'll quit." Certainly, the standard of patient care must be maintained; however, the means of motivating EMTs to meet those standards are dramatically different between paid and volunteer squads.[6,13] Negative motivators, such as pay suspension, extra duties, and demotion, do not apply to volunteers. Instead, personal, positive motivators are tremendously powerful in the volunteer culture.

Pride, expectation, and professionalism are goals of both the EMTs and the medical director. Regular continuing education, skills practice, and oral case simulations with the medical director can be a means to achieving these goals. One-on-one interaction is possible in the rural setting, whereas it may not be feasible in a large urban system. This individual interaction with the medical director is an effective means of assessing knowledge base, protocol familiarity, and thought patterns. It is also a good tool for screening out EMTs who will not succeed in the field. Such sessions clearly establish lines of authority and accountability and make the EMT more personally invested in protecting the medical director's medical license by providing good care.

While maintaining the standards for patient care, it is important to acknowledge the other responsibilities that volunteer EMT organizations have, such as building and equipment maintenance, fund-raising, and squad administration.[1] Stress is becoming recognized more as a significant source of EMT turnover. Incident debriefing by trained peers can be valuable, especially when most of the patients are personally known to the EMTs within the community. Volunteers also have a tremendous sense of dedication, without consideration for time. When in a crisis, they may work endlessly and need to be forceably removed for rest.[6]

Opening the channels of communication can be uncomfortable. Criticism is a two-way process, and the problem with a particular call on the radio may very well be with the physician or the mobile intensive care nurses rather than the

EMTs. In the past, postgraduate physician training in EMS direction has been virtually nonexistent.[11] However, all staff who interact with EMS in a decision-making capacity should be methodically oriented to the operating procedures and protocols, and evaluated regularly for proficiency.

Most rural areas are served at a basic-care level.[16] Advancement of service requires a tremendous commitment. Identifying "essential" skills and medications helps to refine training. Many providers of intermediate levels are allowed to start intravenous fluids but cannot endotracheally intubate; is this a logical expansion?[4] Does the use of pneumatic antishock trousers constitute an essential service?[9] Prospective research is difficult to do in this setting and not enthusiastically carried out by most volunteer EMTs. Unfortunately, the available urban data are not readily applicable to the rural setting.[11,17] Longitudinal retrospective analyses, despite their flaws, can provide useful information on the impact of various skills.

An area can upgrade its level of service more economically by using mixed team configurations, such as a paramedic, an intermediate EMT, and a basic EMT, or by considering one of several tiered response schemes. Within a volunteer squad, EMTs who may not perform well in patient care may have talents that can be directed for the benefit of the squad, such as vehicle maintenance, bookkeeping, organizing fund-raisers, or driving the ambulance.

Summary

Being a rural medical director involves considerable on-site training. Adapting to the culture and the values of the community is essential to success. The profile of emergencies, call volume, and volunteer structure are clearly different from most urban systems. However, there is an opportunity for more individual involvement with each EMT and incredible satisfaction and accomplishment. A QA program can succeed if it is based on these concepts and it becomes an integral part of the EMS program. Then attitudes will change, and the prehospital health-care team will be doing a particular thing, not "for QA," but because "that's how it ought to be done." The high level of intrinsic motivation that most volunteers have is an advantage that rural systems have over urban systems. Because of the smaller number of squad members and the lower call volume, a medical director is able to integrate more personally into the system.

REFERENCES

 1. Adams R: Crisis time for rural EMS, *Firehouse* 12-13, 1991.
 2. Baker SP, Whitfield MA, O'Neill B: Geographic variations in mortality from motor vehicle crashes, *N Engl J Med* 316(22):1384-1387, 1987.
 3. Beck DM: Help wanted (we will train)—a report on the development of volunteer EMS, *J Emerg Med Serv* 13(6):43-49, 1988.
 4. Donovan PJ et al: Prehospital care by EMTs and EMT-Is in a rural setting: prolongation of scene times by ALS procedures, *Ann Emerg Med* 18(5):495-500, 1989.

5. Garnett GF, Hall JE, Johnson MS: *Rural emergency medical services.* In Kuehl AE, editor: *NAEMSP EMS medical directors handbook,* St. Louis, 1989, Mosby—Year Book.
6. Gora JG, Nemerowicz GM: *Emergency squad volunteers—professionalism in unpaid work,* New York, 1985, Praeger Publishers/CBS International Publishing.
7. Grove S: N.C. areas likened to third world, *Raleigh News and Observer,* May 28, 1988.
8. Hopkins RS: Farm equipment injuries in a rural county, 1980 through 1985: the emergency department as a source of data for prevention, *Ann Emerg Med* 18(7):758-762, 1989.
9. Mattox KL et al: Prospective MAST study in 911 patients, *J Trauma* 29(8):1104-1112, 1989.
10. McCallion R, Jaquysh T: Audio tapes: the key to a sound defib program, *J Emerg Med Serv* 15(4):11-13, 1990.
11. Reeder L: The drought in rural EMS, *J Emerg Med Serv* 14(6):42-49, 1989.
12. Swan TH: Recruiting EMS volunteers, *J Emerg Med Serv* 13(6):51-54, 1988.
13. Swan TH: Keeping volunteers in service, *J Emerg Med Serv* 13(6):55-57, 1988.
14. Swor RA, Hoelzer M: A computer-assisted quality assurance audit in a multiprovider EMS system, *Ann Emerg Med* 19(3):286-290, 1990.
15. Swor RA, Krome RL: Administrative support of emergency medical services medical directors: a profile, *Prehospital and Disaster Medicine* 5(1):25-30, 1990.
16. United States Congress, Office of Technology Assessment: *Rural emergency medical services—special report,* OTA-H-445, Washington, D.C., 1989. US Government Printing Office.
17. Waller JA: Urban-oriented methods: failure to solve rural emergency care problems, *JAMA* 226(12):1441-1446, 1973.

14

Quality Assurance in Suburban EMS Systems

Robert A. Swor, D.O.

Quality assurance (QA) throughout the health-care industry is undergoing a dramatic revolution. The emphasis on quality improvement (QI) programs by the Joint Commission on Healthcare Organizations (JCAHO) will doubtlessly change how health care is evaluated and rendered. Prehospital care, with its emphasis on a systems approach, should be fertile soil for this approach to problem solving. The suburban emergency medical services (EMS) environment will continue to hold unique challenges for EMS system leaders who must have an appreciation of the limitations and challenges of the suburban EMS system.

Suburban Environments

Since the days of television's Ozzie and Harriet, suburban life has been a fundamental part of the "American dream." During the 1960s, the population of suburbs increased 33%, whereas the population of cities increased only 1%. The 1980 census documented that 40% of all U.S. citizens lived in the nation's suburbs.[1]

Some disagreement exists as to what actually defines a suburban area. Early definitions by the census bureau identified it as being an area around a central city (greater than a 50,000-person population) where the primary area of employment was the city. As major suburban areas, such as Nassau and Suffolk counties in New York and Orange County in California, developed, it became clear that a suburban area was not necessarily labor-dependent on the central city.

Suburbs are typically nonagricultural areas with low population densities yet are highly populated. They appear to be growing. Southeastern Michigan

140

around Detroit, for example, is projected to increase urbanized land by 40% by the year 2010, with only a 5% increase in population.[23] Suburban regions are characterized by political and economic fragmentation, the result of many independent local governments without a central authority to facilitate central planning. They are typically more affluent than the central city, and key issues in service provision tend to involve the coordination of services rather than the cost.

Initial funding of EMS systems served to aggravate the problems of coordinating EMS in the suburbs. Grants provided for by the EMS Act of 1973 (the 1200 series grants) called for development of 303 EMS regions, each of approximately 750,000 residents, throughout the country. Some of those regions were single cities with large, single-service EMS systems. Most, however, incorporated multiple cities into a single heterogeneous EMS region composed of providers from a number of cities and townships.[11]

Suburban EMS systems are not well characterized. In general, they are complex, with multiple agencies providing care. The actual number of units and personnel available is greater than those of single-service urban systems. Similarly, dispatch is fragmented, with multiple public safety answering points (PSAPs) serving as 9-1-1 answering points.[17] Some suburban cities may be large enough to function as an independent unit and more closely emulate an urban EMS system, even though there is little literature that addresses the "small-city EMS system." This chapter focuses on multiprovider suburban EMS systems.

Issues faced in the evaluation of EMS systems are a microcosm of the problems faced by suburbs as a whole: multiple providers of services; disseminated authority; lack of centralized resources; mistrust of central authority; and demands for confidentiality.

Data Collection and Handling

Coordination of the varied sources for data collection and evaluation is a major logistic burden for the suburban EMS system. Sources of patient care data include standardized EMS run sheets, agency dispatch logs, base-station order sheets, and emergency department and in-patient records. Agreements must be obtained to allow data access (or submission of necessary data) with all these varied organizations. Concrete assurances must be given that confidentiality will be maintained. Centralization of record handling with proper controls for these records is critical for QA program development, but suburban systems will experience increased costs attributed to such collection methods.

Developing Standards for EMS

Few standards have been developed that specifically address a multiprovider, suburban EMS system. National standards that address the care of individual patients apply equally to urban, suburban, and rural systems. Performance standards for training are also similar. Considerations of particular importance in the suburban environment include the process of standard development, the local operational standards, and the need for performance standards that cross municipal boundaries.

The composition of most suburban systems is one of multiple agencies with variable call volumes and often divergent populations and case mix. Because of this diversity, uniform standards are crucial to ensure uniform quality of care within a region. Multiple agencies have unique needs and constraints in their ability to adhere to standards. A broad-based, consensus approach to standard development with exhaustive discussion is, therefore, absolutely vital if standards are to be enforceable throughout the region. Unless this political process is adhered to, retrospective enforcement of standards is doomed to failure. Specific standards, such as training, staff levels, continuing education, and patient care protocols, must all be addressed. In addition, a failure to have appropriate standards in place may serve as a basis for malpractice actions against an EMS system.[13]

Standards for documentation, radio communications, and data collection are often overlooked and should be developed as well. Key data elements of information for radio reports and run sheets should be identified for all cases and specific case types. These standards serve both as a model for orienting new EMTs into the system and for retrospective review of patient care. Such information is included in a medical report manual, which is used in many large systems.

Development of operational standards is complex, because few models of suburban systems exist in the medical literature.[8,11] Suburban regions have diverse characteristics, including high-rise office and apartment buildings and relatively sparsely populated areas within the same region. Proposing uniform standards for response time, such as a 90%, less than 8-minute response, in these systems may be unrealistic. Agreement should be reached on what is locally obtainable for appropriate patient care; strategies then can be devised to meet those standards.

Evaluation of System Components

System- versus Service-Based Review

Evaluation of system components must take place at both the level of the individual service and systemwide. Confidentiality and logistic factors favor the use of in-house, service-based activities to evaluate compliance with standards, performance of invasive procedures, minor incidents, and appropriate documentation. Evaluation by an independent agency must also take place to provide impartial confirmation of standard compliance, review major incidents, and assess system parameters that cross agency boundaries.

Prospective Evaluation

Prospective evaluation of the suburban EMS system is the major means by which quality of care can be ensured. Determining that the components are in place to provide quality EMS care is critically important. It is also logistically less burdensome than other methods of review. Key parameters to review include system structure, key policies and procedures for patient care, standing orders for direct patient care, and credentials of providers at the many different levels of care.

Credentialing of providers is an important task and, to a large extent, dictates the standard of care that is provided in a system. Requirements for paramedics in most systems include initial training requirements and further local training demands. Advanced cardiac life support and basic trauma life support certifications are two of the most common additional requirements. Many systems also require practical or didactic testing at the time of recertification. Documentation of procedural proficiency is required by some large systems. Alameda County, California, and King County, Washington, require a minimum number of intubations to qualify for paramedic recertification. This practice makes particular sense in suburban systems that have a relatively large number of paramedics and advanced life support units (which dilute each individual's procedural expertise) when compared with single-system urban systems.[7,20]

Unfortunately, requirements for basic emergency medical technicians and first responders are not as well defined. The large number of providers and the limited resources of medical control authorities make this task difficult. With the development of automatic defibrillator programs, attention is placed on credentialing standards for these providers. Yet this process needs to extend beyond the care of cardiac arrest victims, who make up only a small percentage of EMS systems' volume.

Interest in EMS dispatch has recently developed nationwide with the realization of its critical role in coordinating EMS care. This is particularly true in suburban systems in which there is often a decentralized system of PSAPs, an area that local municipalities perceive as an important local function. Standards for dispatch of appropriate level of service and medical interrogation of the caller must be developed, although authority for assessing compliance may not be the prerogative of the EMS agency.

Credentialing must also take place for facilities and personnel that provide medical direction and receive emergency patients. Medical directors must have sufficient knowledge and experience regarding emergency care to provide assistance when consulted by radio. They must also be familiar with the capabilities and limitations of the prehospital care setting. California, as an example, requires training in a standard base-station course and certification to provide online medical direction.[19] A secondary benefit of this process is that it allows a concurrent review of field care by a trained provider. Finally, guidelines must exist for a system medical director.

QA for receiving facilities is often beyond the scope of a system's authority and falls to the state health department. Clearly, the system must have destination policies based on the capabilities of its receiving facilities and must monitor whether those facilities are able to provide care consistent with their stated capabilities. A prospective review of the system is the critical starting point to ensure that all components are in place to provide quality care (see Chapter 4).

Concurrent Evaluation

Review of care as it is being provided on scene is the optimal method of ensuring quality medical care. Positive behavior may be reinforced and errors corrected before patient care is affected and bad habits develop. Systems such as Houston's and Pittsburgh's make extensive use of on-scene review (see Chapter 18). This task is resource intensive, however, and suburban systems rarely have the population density to allow frequent on-scene response by a single medical director. Delegation of this function to a field supervisor is more likely to ensure a field presence in this environment.

Alternative methods of concurrent review include review when the patient arrives at the hospital and by online medical direction. The value of online direction for patient care has come under increased scrutiny in recent years. However, it remains a means by which a paramedic's patient evaluation and interpretation of a situation can be reviewed in a contemporaneous fashion. If medical direction is centralized (which is uncommon in suburban systems), concurrent evaluation of the system is done on an ongoing basis. For decentralized systems, monitoring of radio transmissions by trained medical personnel may serve a similar (albeit expensive and redundant) task. This method of review requires that radio communication occur, which may not be the case in important instances (e.g., patient refusal of care).

Although it is not absolutely concurrent, feedback on field care rendered is best reviewed at the time the patient arrives at the receiving facility. Field impressions can then be compared with physician evaluation and with other clinical data. This requires the receiving physician to have the time and interest to critically review the prehospital care rendered and to give feedback. In systems with multiple receiving hospitals, a coordinated evaluation by receiving physicians can be a logistic nightmare. Many systems make liberal use of EMS system review sheets, which are widely distributed and may be completed by any person in a system when a concern is raised regarding patient care. This method does not, however, serve as a substitute for a systematic evaluation of care.

Retrospective Review

Retrospective review of care is what one typically thinks of when QA is discussed. Realistically, it is a small part of a QA program and is probably the most time-consuming and the least valuable. Information gathered retrospectively is most likely to be incomplete, and the greater the time gap between the review and the care rendered, the more likely important information will be

Possible Explicit Parameters
for Review

All field providers

Trauma scenes > 15 minutes
  Refusal of transportation
  Immediate life and limb threats
  Multicasualty incidents
  Patient deterioration en route to hospital
  Communication failure
  Equipment failure
  Cardiac arrest and automatic defibrillator use

Cognitive-technical skills

Assessment compared with emergency department discharge diagnosis
  Intubation attempt
  EKG interpretation
  Communication skills
  Time to defibrillation—paramedics and EMT-basics

Dispatch

Time through dispatch (98% < 2 minutes, e.g., Fresno Co., Calif.)[19]
  Identification of critical cases (those requiring transport to hospital with lights and sirens)[20]

Online medical control

Availability
  Identified
  Appropriate for system
  Efficient

lacking. Methodology of review and definitions of terms have been discussed previously.

Coordinating a comprehensive review of a system with multiple providers is a daunting task that requires access to records, logistic support, and most importantly, political support from the providers being reviewed. The review of multiple agencies assumes that comparisons are made between agencies. Assurances must be given that findings are treated in a confidential fashion.

A base-line review must be performed to evaluate the areas in which a QA program would be most effective. Some authors advocate a 100% chart review,[19] although this, too, is time-consuming and inefficient. Each system has preexisting areas that system members can readily identify as areas for review. A laundry list of areas targeted for explicit, objective initial review can be constructed using standards developed locally or nationally (see box on page

145). Discussion must then ensue regarding local system priorities to ensure appropriate use of resources and generate systemwide agreement on the value of the review. For instance, suburban EMS systems commonly lack the volume of penetrating trauma seen in urban EMS systems, and providers have less experience with critically injured trauma patients. A review of trauma scene times and procedures might be appropriate.

The focus of retrospective review must extend beyond field care. If in keeping with most suburban systems there are multiple providers of online medical direction, monitoring must occur to ensure consistency, availability, and appropriateness of medical direction rendered.[18] This can be accomplished by online monitoring by the medical director or the designee or by review of run tapes. Similarly, if there are multiple agencies providing medical dispatch, the accuracy and timeliness of their activities should be monitored.

Prioritization of QA activities is an important issue that requires substantial attention. Reviews should be of limited duration and not run concurrently. Morale is significantly affected by the bombardment of paperwork and the perception that ''big brother is always watching.''

Outcome measures must also be applied to assess function of the entire system. Most commonly, cardiac arrest or trauma mortality rates are used as parameters. These evaluations are complex and expensive (see Chapters 16 and 21).

Facilitating Change

The true value of a successful QA program is to objectively identify and quantify areas for improvement. This emphasis on QI pervades industries in the United States and is being widely implemented in the health-care industry. Key features of QI include a philosophy that employees work diligently to perform their duties, an emphasis that faulty *processes* must be improved if care is to improve, a commitment to quality from senior management, and an empowerment of caregivers to improve the system of care (see Chapter 6). Structural components of a system necessary to facilitate improvement include good communications throughout the system, reinforcement of positive behavior, and involvement of caregivers at all levels of the QA program. The issue of adequate communication is a particularly troubling one for the decentralized multiprovider, suburban EMS system.

Education

Traditionally, education has been used to change behavior. A QA program produces an educational program with vitality because it develops material for relevant training. Tape review sessions, which are well received by EMS providers, are a classic example. The National Association of EMS Physicians, for example, advocates that tape review sessions be a regular part of a dispatch QA program.[13] However, significant obstacles still exist to good EMS education. In the suburban environment the number of agencies and providers complicates efforts to ensure consistent relevant education based on QA findings. In the northern Chicago area, for instance, the EMS authority coordinates in excess of 60 continuing education programs per month.[17] To address this issue, innovative techniques (such as systemwide computer bulletin boards and EMS continuing education cable television programs) have been tested. The issue of consistent and accessible provider education on a continuing basis must be addressed for a QA program to have any impact.

Hospital-based Clinical Rotations

Most EMS clinical skills are best taught within the confines of the hospital. The varied nature of EMS call volume limits adequate exposure to individual clinical problems. Retraining in specific skills, such as intravenous technique, emergency deliveries, pediatric assessments, and endotracheal intubation, may all be refined during hospital clinical exposure. Unfortunately, the sheer volume of providers prevents hospitals from being able to offer such training on a consistent basis. Endotracheal intubation especially is a skill in which access to training is limited. The system medical director must aggressively pursue these training sites if procedural deficiencies are identified by the QA process.

Provider Quality Assurance Participation

Participation by auditors in peer review has been widely recognized as a valuable technique for educating physicians regarding important QA issues and forcing them to evaluate their own practice.[2,24] We have reviewed paramedic peer review auditing in our own system and have found it to be a valuable technique in educating paramedics regarding their own practice.[28] It also has served as a valuable adjunct in an ongoing QA program, facilitating a daily review of patient care and identifying trends in field care and documentation.[29] This program has been most effective as an initial explicit review and requires the ongoing participation of the physician medical director to further evaluate cases and investigate issues raised by paramedic auditors. QI programs in industry and health care demand an active involvement by caregivers in process evaluation to improve care.

Physician Input

The role of the physician in effecting change is crucial to any EMS system.[16,25] His effectiveness can be maximized if that role is perceived as being a patient advocate and educator. This "white-hat" approach is well received by providers, especially if the physician is knowledgeable regarding the limitations of field care.

Management Issues

EMS agency management must be an ongoing partner in the QA program. Management must be in agreement with program goals and must be apprised of pertinent findings and issues. Support for interventions, including continuing education, clinical training, and participation in auditing, must be ongoing. Specific instances that demand management involvement are cases in which disciplinary action, retraining, or outright dismissal may be contemplated. Many interventions will have been previously proscribed under employment contracts or union agreements. A more complete discussion regarding these issues is included in Chapter 10.

Summary

QA activities in the suburban EMS system are severely hampered unless a central agency exists to coordinate data collection, funding, and communication between agencies and field providers. Systems must successfully address these issues to maximize their efforts.

Some regions (e.g., San Francisco, King County, Washington, and Burbank, California) have developed organizations for the evaluation of prehospital care. These organizations greatly reduce the logistic impediments to quality EMS care.

A clear goal of any QA program is improved patient care. Yet a surprising outcome of QA activities reported in one survey is an improved relationship with street EMS providers.[12] Some organizations support QA activities for this reason alone. Problems peculiar to the suburban EMS environment include the relatively large number of providers for population base, the difficulty in coordinating education and communication, and the lack of standards specific for suburban systems.

REFERENCES

1. Baldassare M: *Trouble in paradise*. In: *The suburban transformation in America,* New York, 1986, Columbia University Press.
2. Berwick D: Sounding board: continuous improvement as an ideal in health care, *N Engl J Med* 320:53-56, 1989.
3. Berwick, DM, Godfrey AB, Roessner J: *Curing health care: new strategies for quality improvement,* San Francisco, 1990, Jossey-Bass.
4. Braun O, McCallion R, Fazackerley J: Characteristics of midsized urban EMS systems, *Ann Emerg Med* 19(5):536-546, 1990.
5. Champion HR et al: MTOS: establishing national norms for trauma care, *J Trauma* 3(11):1356-1365, 1990.
6. Clawson JJ, Dernocoeur K: *Principles of emergency medical dispatch,* Englewood Cliffs, NJ, 1988, The Brady Co.
7. Eisenberg MS et al: Cardiac arrest and resuscitation: a tale of 29 cities, *Ann Emerg Med* 19(2):179-186, 1990.
8. Eitel DR et al: Out of hospital cardiac arrest: a six year experience in a suburban-rural system, *Ann Emerg Med* 17(8):808-812, 1988.

9. Kallsen GW: *The nuts and bolts of EMS quality assurance,* Presented at ACEP Scientific Assembly, New Orleans, 1988.

10. Kallsen G, Nabors MO: The use of priority medical dispatch to distinguish between high and low risk patients, *Ann Emerg Med* 19(4):458-459 (abstract).

11. Lilja GP, Swor RA: *Emergency medical services.* In Tintinalli JE, editor: *Emergency medicine: a comprehensive study guide,* ed 2, New York, 1988, McGraw-Hill.

12. Maio RF, Bronken T: *Quality assurance in emergency medical services: report of a survey,* Presented at Michigan EMS Expo, Lansing, Mich, 1990.

13. National Association of Emergency Medical Physicians. *Draft position paper on emergency medical dispatching,*

14. Overton DT: A computer-assisted emergency department chart audit, *Ann Emerg Med* 16(1):68-72, 1987.

15. Pepe et al: The impact of intense physician supervision on the effectiveness of an EMS system, *Ann Emerg Med* 17(7):752, 1988 (abstract).

16. Pepe PE, Stewart RD: Role of the physician in the prehospital setting, *Ann Emerg Med* 15:1480-1483, 1986.

17. Ryan J, Zydlo S, Bruns B: Personal communications, 1990.

18. Pointer J: The advanced life support base hospital audit for medical control in an emergency medical services system, *Ann Emerg Med* 16:557-560, 1987.

19. Rottman SJ, Fitzgerald-Westby K: A method for reviewing radio-telemetry paramedic calls, *Ann Emerg Med* 10:36-38, 1981.

20. Ryan J: *Quality assurance in emergency medical services.* In Kuehl AE, editor: *EMS medical directors handbook,* St. Louis, 1989, Mosby-Year Book.

21. Shackford SR, Cooper GF, Eastman AB: Quality in a trauma system: medical audit committee: composition, cost and results, *J Trauma* 27:866-875, 1987.

22. Soler JM et al: The ten-year malpractice experience of a large urban EMS system, *Ann Emerg Med* 14(10):982-985, 1985.

23. Southeastern Michigan Council of Governments, 1990.

24. Stair TO: Quality assurance, *Emerg Med Clin North Am* 5(1):41-54, 1987.

25. Stewart RD: Medical direction in emergency medical services: the role of the physician, *Emerg Med Clin North Am* 5(1):119-132, 1987.

26. Stewart R et al: A computer assisted quality assurance system for an emergency medical service, *Ann Emerg Med* 14(1):25-29, 1985.

27. Stout JL: *System financing.* In Roush WR, editor: *Principles of EMS systems: a comprehensive text for physicians,* Dallas, 1989, American College of Emergency Physicians.

28. Swor RA, Bocka JJ: *A paramedic peer review audit,* Poster presented at annual meeting National Association of EMS Physicians, Houston, 1989.

29. Swor RA, Hoelzer MH: A computer-assisted quality assurance audit in a multi-provider EMS system, *Ann Emerg Med* 19(3):286-290, 1990.

15

Air Medical Transport

Nicholas Benson, M.D.

Medical Direction

Air medical transport quality assurance (QA) programs require the same two foundations necessary in all other areas of health care: the integral involvement of a physician and a comprehensive approach to the review of all aspects of the service. Although the medical care may be delivered by flight nurses, emergency medical technician–paramedics (EMT-Ps), or others, direct participation by physicians is still essential. Experts from other disciplines should assist to provide an integrated quality review. For example, individuals with expertise in communications should handle that portion of the QA program, whereas pilots and mechanics should carry the responsibility for the aviation portion.

In every significant aspect, medical direction *is* QA. Online and offline medical direction involves the supervision and review by physicians regarding the quality of care that an air medical service delivers. Thus enthusiastic and committed medical direction is a necessary component.

It is vital to remember that QA is a problem-solving tool. QA can take vague problems and pull them into focus to make them concrete and specific. It can uncover occult problems through data that clearly indicate a defect. Resolutions for problems can be developed through QA action plans and evaluated at reassessment intervals.

The Plan

A written QA plan is essential. Starting an air medical QA program without a plan would be like setting out for a drive from Miami to Seattle without looking at a road map: you might ultimately arrive at your destination, but the trip would be circuitous and fraught with otherwise preventable problems.

The written QA plan should contain several elements. It should briefly describe the purpose of the air medical service and the QA program itself. It should specify the lines of authority for QA, both within the service and in reporting to the sponsoring body. The plan should list the specific responsibilities

150

for various persons in the air medical service involved with the QA activities. A schedule of specific review and evaluation activities should be included, although this is subject to change. Finally, the plan should be reviewed, renewed, and updated on an annual basis to keep it current.

Ten Steps of Quality Assurance

The Joint Commission on Accreditation of Healthcare Organizations (JCAHO) has developed a "road map" for planning and implementing a QA program. The 10 steps of this road map lay a strong foundation for QA activities in any setting; they are as applicable to air medical transport as they are to inpatient units.[10]

This approach parallels methods that emphasize review of structure, process, and outcome, as discussed elsewhere in this text. All air medical QA programs need to incorporate elements of structure, process, and outcome by following the 10-step approach. However, the most important of these three elements is outcome. The QA program should place heavy emphasis on determining whether the service delivers the desired, optimal outcome to its consumers. In patient care terms, this generally means prevention of morbidity and mortality, although from the aviation and communications aspect, it might mean an absence of crashes or accidents, as well as consistent, clear radio communication with the aircraft.

1. The JCAHO's 10 steps begin by assigning specific responsibilities to individuals. These responsibilities should be clearly laid out in the QA plan but also need to be explained to the specific individuals involved and to the entire staff. It is important for everyone to have an understanding of the roles that the key players have, as well as their accountability. The number and types of individuals involved may vary from service to service, but generally they include the medical director, the service's manager, a medical team member, a communication specialist, a pilot, the service's education and safety officers, and the administrator for the sponsoring institution, be it a hospital or a public-service agency.

2. A scope-of-care statement should be written. This is simply a complete written inventory of what the service does. It defines what aspects of care need to be reviewed, as well as specifies how this service differs from other health-care delivery services in the region. A sample scope of care for a fictitious air medical service, LifeFlight XYZ, is offered in the sidebar on page 152.

3. Once the type of service is described, the important aspects of care are specified. This list should include specific elements of the service that most need to be performed well. For a comprehensive QA approach to an air medical service, this list should include patient care, communications, and aviation components. For example, this might include airway control for scene response patients with head injuries, prompt recognition of ventricular dysrhythmias in patients with cardiac illness, quality control checks on the helipad's in-ground fuel system, incidence of flights aborted because of weather for each pilot, and adherence to "flight-following" communications every 10 minutes.

LifeFlight XYZ
Scope of Care

As a regional air medical transport provider, this fictitious service offers emergency medical air transport services 24 hours a day to patients with all types of critical illnesses or injuries. Using a helicopter ambulance and a fixed-wing ambulance, the service meets a broad range of needs and transports patients up to thousands of miles. The service is prepared to perform interhospital transports, respond to trauma scenes, or in extreme situations, provide emergency transportation for medications or other treatment modalities.

In its role as a regional service the service is closely integrated with all of the community hospitals in its rural referral area and the regional ground EMS authority, although it is wholly sponsored by Hospital XYZ.

The staff is composed of 16 fully trained critical care flight nurses, 6 pilots, a mechanic, and a medical director. Each flight is staffed by two flight nurses and a pilot. Online medical control is continuously provided by radio or telephone for all transports. When the flight nurses are not actively engaged in flight duties, they are available to provide spot help in the sponsor hospital.

Hospital XYZ is a regional teaching medical center, is fully integrated with XYZ University School of Medicine, and contains 750 beds. It has specialty critical care services in the following areas: cardiac intensive, cardiac surgery intensive, medical intensive, surgical intensive, neurosurgical intensive, pediatric intensive, pulmonary intensive, and neonatal intensive. It is designated as a regional level-I trauma center.

The service fulfills the following responsibilities:

1. Provides a fully trained and staffed critical care transport staff and environment at all times for critically ill or injured patients.
2. Provides stabilization for patients at the referral site prior to loading the patient onto the aircraft for transport.
3. Maintains a comprehensive preventive maintenance program to ensure maximal availability of the aircraft.
4. Evaluates its operations constantly to review the safety of procedures and policies to provide the safest transport environment possible.
5. Provides periodic refresher training for all staff members in their respective disciplines.

Common patient problems cared for include the following: blunt trauma to the torso, closed head injury, spinal cord injury, acute myocardial infarction with pump failure, acute respiratory failure, septic shock, pediatric respiratory emergencies, and premature neonates with respiratory insufficiency.

Procedures frequently performed include the following: invasive airway maneuvers, establishing peripheral and central intravenous lines, maintenance of multiple intravenous medication infusions, mechanical ventilation, and intensive vital sign monitoring.

This listing of the important aspects of care parallels prior QA doctrines that called for the creation of standards of care. These standards, or important aspects, are the cornerstones of the air medical service. They define expectations of behavior and performance. This is especially true for the human components but also may be applied to the equipment and the supplies. These standards may be developed using the opinions of the service's own staff, since they have an established local expertise in air medical transport.

Alternatively, external sources may be reviewed for relevant standards. These external sources might include a regional EMS council, a state EMS regulatory agency, the advanced trauma life support course,[3] the advanced cardiac life support course,[4] pediatric advanced life support courses,[5] and other national organizations, such as the National Flight Nurses Association and the Association of Air Medical Services. These standards must be written in objective terms so that they lend themselves to measurable analysis. The important aspects of care must be periodically reanalyzed and refined as the air medical service and the QA program mature.

4. The list of important aspects of care should be categorized as high risk, problem prone, or high volume. Of course, any particular important aspect may fit into one or more categories. This categorization offers a perspective for prioritizing the review of the important aspects. Since no air medical service can hope to tackle the entire list of important aspects at one time, especially at the initiation of a QA program, this categorization should suggest the most urgent areas for initial review. For example, in many air medical services this categorization leads directly to initiation of QA activities that include airway stabilization maneuvers, flight-following communications, and aircraft safety at scene responses. A sample listing of important aspects of care, including categorization, can be found in the box on page 154.

Following categorization, clinical indicators can be derived using the important aspects of care. This is simply a restatement of the important aspects of care into statements of expected behavior. These statements should be in objective and measurable terms that reflect current scientific or behavioral knowledge. For example, "airway control for scene response patients with head injuries" becomes "head-injured patients with Glasgow coma scores of 6 or less will be intubated at the scene." The indicators should be reviewed by the staff of the air medical service so that the staff can agree on their importance.

To illustrate this development, LifeFlight XYZ has decided that an important aspect of care is the stabilization of trauma patients at scene responses. This has been rephrased to a standard that states that "multiple-trauma patients will receive spinal immobilization and airway management at the scene." Two clinical indicators follow from this standard: 1) Multiple-trauma patients with significant head and/or neck trauma, or decreased mental status, or neck pain, or acute upper extremity neurologic deficits will undergo complete spinal immobilization. 2) Multiple-trauma patients with respiratory distress, or significant hypovolemia, or head injuries, or major chest trauma will undergo airway stabilization.

Potential Important Aspects of Care for an Air Medical Transport Service

Scene care

- Trauma patient stabilization (high risk)
- Management of cervical spine injuries (high risk)
- Invasive airway management (problem prone, high risk)
- On-scene medical control (problem prone)
- Landing zone preparation (high risk, problem prone)
- Intravenous fluid administration (high volume)

Referring institution interaction

- Initial information gathering (problem prone)
- Assessment of patient (high risk, high volume)
- Packaging of patient (problem prone, high volume)
- Interaction with referring physician (high volume)
- Encountering patients with problems other than anticipated (high risk, problem prone)

Patient care in transport

- Monitoring of vital signs, airway, fluids, and medications (high risk)
- Communication with medical control (problem prone)
- Cardiopulmonary resuscitation (high risk, problem prone)
- Transports to hospital other than sponsor institution (problem prone)

Patient management protocols

- Cardiac dysrhythmias (high risk, high volume)
- Airway management and mechanical ventilation (high risk, high volume)
- Multiple trauma (high risk, high volume)
- Combative patients (high risk, problem prone)
- Circulatory failure (high risk, high volume)
- Pediatric respiratory failure (high risk)

The four steps described above result in a ranking of items that require review from the entire breadth of the air medical service.

5. The fifth step is to decide what level of compliance is required. Is the particular behavior (i.e., the clinical indicator) so important as to require compliance 100% of the time? Or is 75% a more reasonable goal? In JCAHO terminology this is referred to as the *threshold for evaluation*. The threshold is a specific percentage of compliance. If this threshold is not reached, an investigation is then undertaken to determine the reasons for noncompliance.

Many new QA programs set thresholds for their indicators at 100%. This is an admirable goal, but frequently unattainable. It is vital to be realistic in setting a threshold, while always leaving some room for improvement. Human nature and other unpredictable factors always impact an air medical service. Allowance for these inevitable errors must be made, as long as the allowance does not jeopardize the patient's outcome or the staff's safety. Thresholds can be established by staff consensus or derived from clinical literature or national associations.

6. The sixth and seventh JCAHO points deal with the process of evaluating the quality of the air medical service provided. It is at this point that the QA personnel actually begin to gather data. To collect data before knowing how and where they would be applied is a waste of time. In gathering data the decision must be made whether to review 100% of relevant flights or to review a sample. The more frequent an instance occurs, the less necessary it is to review every instance. For example, to monitor compliance with a flight-following protocol in a program with 150 transports a month requires only a sample. On the other hand a review of medication dosages in pediatric cardiac arrests necessitates gathering data on every pediatric cardiac arrest for most air medical services.

Sources of data are varied. The flight record is an obvious resource. However, the emergency department record and inpatient records are also helpful, as is the emergency department logbook, the maintenance records, and the communication center records. Recording tapes may be of some use. Evaluations of the patients on arrival at the receiving hospital may also be helpful. Finally, questionnaires to patients and to other air medical service consumers may offer new ideas, as can incident reports and complaints. The most immediate source of data is the concurrent review. Placing an extra staff member on the aircraft, at the scene landing zone, or in the communications center offers an extremely useful opportunity to gather data as the flight actually occurs.

Of course, the medical director cannot gather all these data by himself. Consistent and enthusiastic support is needed from medical, communications, and aviation personnel. This support can be assisted through a monitoring calendar that specifies the time each month that data will be gathered.

7. After the data are collected, it is then time to evaluate the data. Generally, this is as simple as comparing the rate of compliance with the threshold for evaluation. If the compliance exceeds the threshold, then no evaluation need be done. However, if the compliance rate fails to meet the threshold, then all instances in which the indicator was not met need to be reviewed.

In conducting this evaluation it may be wise to look at data from the entire service. Alternatively, some problems call for evaluation of data from just one shift, or from one day of the week, or from one portion of the service's staff. This evaluation process varies from service to service and from indicator to indicator. The most essential aspect of the evaluation is that it be conducted in an objective fashion that is based on current knowledge. QA should never be used as a "witch hunt."

8. In its eighth point the JCAHO's approach forms an action plan based on evaluation of the data. The action plan should include the following components: clear specification of the problem, identification of who or what behavior is to change to resolve the problem, notation of the time table for expected

change, specification of the individual responsible for effecting the change, what the change in behavior is to include, and when the indicator will be evaluated again. Occasionally, the evaluation reveals a problem that is beyond the influence of the air medical service. At that time the action plan should specify how assistance from external resources will be rallied to increase compliance. Whenever appropriate, the lessons learned from the QA evaluation and the action plan should be incorporated into the continuing-education calendar for the staff.

9. Following the implementation of the action plan the problem is reassessed after a specified interval. It is absolutely vital to determine whether the behavior improved to see if the action plan was successful. If the action did not result in the expected improvement, then a new action plan should be developed.

10. The tenth step involves reporting the QA results to the appropriate parties. This sharing of results is essential for the success of QA activities. However, reports must be handled in a confidential manner. For many QA programs this means that a verbal report is given at meetings, and the official record of the results is filed in a file labeled "confidential." Copies of results and reports generally should not be taken from meetings by individuals. Peer-review statutes in each state offer specific guidelines for maintaining confidentiality and limiting discovery if legal action should occur. These QA results should be shared at staff meetings, board meetings of the governing body, medical advisory council meetings, and other appropriate functions.

Sample Quality Assurance Activities

Missed Esophageal Intubations

One common concern of physicians involved with emergency patient care is the possibility of a missed esophageal intubation. The medical director of LifeFlight XYZ has seen two unresponsive patients this month that the flight team brought in with the endotracheal tube placed unknowingly in the esophagus. This ties in directly with the important aspect of care labeled "airway management (high risk)." A possible standard of care for this situation is that "unresponsive patients will have their airways secured via either endotracheal or nasotracheal intubation." (Individual physicians may vary slightly in their approach to airway stabilization in unresponsive patients. This is merely an example.) Three clinical indicators are possible for this problem:

1. For every patient with endotracheal or nasotracheal intubation, the EMT-P documents in the flight record the quality of breath sounds at the five basic auscultation points. Threshold for evaluation: 95%.
2. Whenever the flight nurse is not certain that the endotracheal or nasotracheal tube is in the trachea, the tube is removed at once. Reintubation may be attempted again. Threshold for evaluation: 100%.

3. EMT-Ps must perform at least two intubations every six months. These may be done in the field, the ED, the OR, or the practice lab. Threshold for evaluation: 90%.

As the data are collected from each of these indicators, the medical director and the service's QA coordinator can try to determine if the deficiency in intubation is a problem common to the entire flight team or whether it involves only specific individuals. Note that the clinical indicators listed above attempt to specify how the technician should know where the tube is located, what to do if the technician is not sure where the tube is located, and how the technician can try to maintain his skill proficiency.

Problems with Intravenous Lines

Many of the cardiac patients flown by LifeFlight XYZ are on numerous intravenous medication infusions. This morass of intravenous tubing, coupled with cardiac monitor leads and other electronic leads, consistently contributes to line tangling and to confusion. The medical director senses that a significant number of intravenous lines on patients are either dislodged or infiltrated on patient arrival at the receiving hospital. This correlates with the important aspect of care of "starting and maintaining intravenous lines (high volume)." An appropriate standard of care would be "When intravenous lines are started on patients, they shall remain patent and capable of delivering fluid and medications." The following three clinical indicators could be used to measure compliance of behavior with this standard:

1. Flight nurses should successfully start intravenous lines en route in appropriate patients. Threshold for evaluation: 80% (success rate for en route starts).
2. Intravenous lines started in the field are patent and functional on the patient's arrival at the receiving hospital. Threshold for evaluation: 90%.
3. Flight nurses perform at least two intravenous line placements per month, whether in the field or in the hospital. Threshold for evaluation: 90%.

The thresholds in this case have been set at a reasonable level, based on a consensus developed at a staff meeting. They recognize that intravenous lines will never be perfect; some infiltration and dislodging is bound to occur. The thresholds also recognize that there will be occasional problems with attempts to start intravenous lines in a moving aircraft. This realistic approach should help establish a standard for the service, as well as uncover potential areas requiring remedial work.

Scene Response Use

Over the past few months the medical director for LifeFlight XYZ has received comments from her colleagues that some patients flown in from scene responses to the receiving trauma center are discharged home from the emergency department. Of course, this raises her concern over the appropriateness of triage criteria used to request LifeFlight XYZ for scene responses. This falls under the important aspect of care of "appropriate use for scene responses (problem prone)." The standard of care might be "Use of the helicopter ambulance for scene responses follows triage criteria approved by the Region Q EMS Advisory Council." The following three clinical indicators might be developed:

1. Trauma patients have a Champion trauma score of 12 or less, or a Glasgow coma score of 8 or less, or a major body system injury. Threshold for evaluation: 80%.
2. Adult patients have one or more of the following vital sign abnormalities: systolic blood pressure less than 90; heart rate less than 60 or greater than 120; respiratory rate less than 10 or more than 30; or unresponsive to verbal stimuli. Threshold for evaluation: 85%.
3. Stable patients who are readily accessible by ground advanced life support services are not to be transported by helicopter from scene responses. Threshold for evaluation: 85%.

Of course, these triage criteria will vary somewhat from locale to locale, as they don't take into account the question of distance from the scene to the receiving trauma center.

Utilization Review

As the air medical transport profession matures, its accountability increases in a variety of ways. One of the major areas requiring increased accountability is the appropriate utilization of emergency air transport services for critically ill and injured patients. Whereas QA evaluates the quality of services rendered, utilization review analyzes whether the patients truly needed the services they were given. Both QA and utilization review programs must integrate patient care and operational indicators to provide a comprehensive approach.

In utilization review it is important to look for trends and patterns, not to overly scrutinize individual flights. Thresholds for evaluation for utilization review are best determined by an individual air medical service, because the regional factors that impact utilization vary. These variances may depend on topography, population density, distribution of appropriate receiving hospitals, and availability of other EMS transport services.

A variety of utilization review criteria are available today for air medical professionals to adapt to local situations. The Quality Assurance Committee of the Association of Air Medical Services has developed a resource document that includes 10 generic utilization review criteria.[6] Organizations in North Carolina, Connecticut, and Massachusetts have developed utilization criteria that are used for services based within their own geographic borders.[7,9,12]

Administrators of all air medical transport services should be involved with utilization review today. With technology as expensive as air ambulances, there is significant potential for abuse. The presence or absence of abuse can really only be determined by cautious review. This review is probably best undertaken by a health-care professional who is external to the air medical service. For a hospital-based service this may mean enlisting the assistance of a nurse or a medical records professional in the hospital's QA office.

Commission on Accreditation of Air Medical Services

In the late 1980s air medical professionals across the nation noticed increasing divergence in the quality of patient care and the safety of the operational approach of certain programs. As a result, seven national organizations with long-standing interests in air medical transport pooled their resources to create the Commission on Accreditation of Air Medical Services (CAAMS). The purpose of this commission was to create a separate nonprofit corporation for the development and implementation of a national voluntary accreditation process for private and public air medical services.

During the first two years of the commission a total of 13 member organizations have joined: the American Academy of Pediatrics, the American Association of Respiratory Care, the American College of Emergency Physicians, the American College of Surgeons Committee on Trauma, the Association of Air Medical Services, the National Association of Air Medical Communication Specialists, the National Association of EMS Physicians, the National Association of Neonatal Nurses, the National Association of State EMS Directors, the National EMS Pilots Association, the National Flight Nurses Association, the National Flight Paramedics Association, and the Professional Aeromedical Transport Association.

The commission has recently implemented its accreditation process, which emphasizes quality assurance and improvement, safe air operations, proper education for all team members, and appropriate equipment for the aircraft and ground team members. The commission is dedicated to assisting programs demonstrate that they provide quality patient care in a safe air transport environment.

Summary

As physicians become involved with or upgrade their QA and utilization review programs, it is important to remember that these should not be seen as being simply paper exercises. They can enable the physician to deliver a higher quality of care in a safer, more appropriate environment. Further, these programs should not be used as a means of identifying individuals for denigration or punishment. They must be conducted in a professional, objective manner to garner support from the professionals within the service.

It is also important to provide QA and utilization review programs that cover all aspects of the air medical service. Without a comprehensive approach, the potential for undiscovered problems will continue.

Reviews of the services rendered can provide substantive motivation for change and offer an effective tool for solving problems. They must be carried out with proactive communication so that all professionals involved with the air medical service are aware and supportive. By demonstrating the high quality of services rendered and by unveiling occult problems, the medical director can use QA and utilization review to increase the morale of the staff and to upgrade the level of the services provided.

REFERENCES

1. Air-medical Crew National Standard Curriculum: *Instructor manual,* Pasadena, Calif, 1988, ASHBEAMS.
2. American Academy of Pediatrics Committee on Hospital Care: Guidelines for air and ground transportation of pediatric patients, *Pediatrics* 78(5):943-950, 1986.
3. American College of Surgeons Committee on Trauma: *Advanced trauma life support course for physicians instructor manual,* Chicago, 1989, American College of Surgeons.
4. American Heart Association: *Textbook of advanced cardiac life support,* Dallas, 1987, American Heart Association.
5. American Heart Association, American Academy of Pediatrics: *Textbook of pediatric advanced life support,* Dallas, 1988, American Heart Association.
6. Association of Air Medical Services Quality Assurance Committee: AAMS resource document for air medical quality assurance programs, *J Air Med Trans* 9(8):23-26, 1990.
7. Blumen IJ, Gordon RS: Taking to the skies, *Emergency* 36-37, 1989.
8. Eastes L, Jacobson J, editors: *Quality assurance in air medical transport,* Orem, Utah, 1990, WordPerfect Publishing Company.
9. Gabram SGA, Jacobs LM: The impact of emergency medical helicopters on prehospital care. *Emerg Med Clin North Am* 8(1):85-102, 1990.
10. Joint Commission on Accreditation of Healthcare Organizations: *Agenda for change update: news from the Joint Commission* 1(1):3, 1987.
11. U.S. Department of Transportation National Highway Traffic Safety Administration, American Medical Association Commission on Emergency Medical Services: *Air ambulance guidelines,* ed 2, 1986, The Department and The Association.
12. Williams K, Aghababian R, Shaughnessy M: Statewide helicopter utilization review: the Massachusetts experience, *J Air Med Trans* 9(9):14-23, 1990.

16

Trauma System Quality Assurance

Brenda Bruns, M.D.

The previous chapters in this text have discussed the structure and function of an effective quality assurance (QA) program in an emergency medical services (EMS) system. This chapter focuses on the issues that are unique to trauma system QA, the components necessary for the development of an effective trauma audit process, and the costs and sources of funding for trauma QA.

Trauma is one of the major health-care problems in the United States today. It is the leading cause of death in persons under 44 years old and the fourth leading cause of death in the general population. The annual cost of accidental injury exceeds $118 billion.[6] Trauma systems have been designed and developed to address this problem. In addition to providing definitive treatment of seriously injured patients, trauma systems manage and/or oversee public-education and injury-prevention programs and prehospital, in-hospital, and rehabilitative patient care.[20]

Regionalization of trauma care has been in existence in parts of the United States for more than a decade.[11] Processes for system design and trauma-center designation have been well described, and the efficacy of trauma systems in reducing preventable deaths as a result of injury has been well supported in the literature.[19] Regionalization of trauma care has involved improvements in all aspects of trauma patient care: transport, response capability, prehospital care, destination and triage guidelines, and designation of trauma centers.[11]

In spite of the positive results of trauma systems, less than half of all states have initiated the process. This reluctance may be because of widespread fundamental problems in existing trauma systems, such as lack of consistent triage criteria, overdesignation of trauma centers, the high cost of extensive human and physical resource allocation, and inadequate system monitoring. Additionally, a lack of trauma data has hindered the development of effective injury-prevention programs and the evaluation of the quality of care trauma patients receive.[6] Yet a comprehensive and effective trauma QA program can mitigate many of these problems. By monitoring and assessing the quality, efficacy, and cost of trauma care from moment of injury to definitive disposition, optimal care will be delivered and the existence of the trauma system justified. Collection, collation, and evaluation of data allow better management and allocation of resources and identify and support the necessity for alterations of the system.

The goal of high-quality trauma care is best attained by designing a QA system with strong prospective, concurrent, and retrospective components. Prospective activities set the standards clearly so that the trauma centers and other system participants know the meaning of their commitment. Data derived from concurrent and retrospective audits provide individual and facility evaluations that enable the trauma system oversight agency and system participants to determine if policies, procedures and contractual agreements are being upheld. The American College of Emergency Physicians (ACEP) and many states with trauma systems recognize the EMS agency (EMSA) as the appropriate oversight agency. Hence, for the remainder of this chapter the term EMSA will be used to represent any oversight agency. If the oversight agency is *not* the EMSA it is important to define the relationships between the EMSA and the oversight body and between the EMSA and the other trauma system participants and to define the EMSA's role in the trauma QA process.

Data derived from QA provide proof to all system participants of the necessity for implementing recommended changes or improvements. They can also be used to identify trauma-specific costs that allow trauma centers to design budgets and support funding needs. Descriptive statistics, such as overtriage and undertriage rates, allow better allocation of resources. Participation of system members on audit committees, where individual cases and system statistics are reviewed and compared to local and national norms, provides motivation for improvement by way of peer pressure, interfacility competition, and education.

The political struggles of trauma systems begin with the decisions to establish a trauma system, to designate specific hospitals as trauma centers, and to identify by way of field triage protocols certain patients as trauma-center candidates; they continue through the process of system monitoring and evaluation. The challenge for the EMSA is to diplomatically use its authority to produce the best trauma system possible. A solidly constructed, well-planned QA system is itself the most likely method for accomplishing the goals of QA: closure of the "feedback loop" and improvement in the quality of patient care.

The following sections provide a detailed description of the steps necessary for developing such a QA system.

Structure: Prospective Components of Quality Assurance

The ACEP describes 11 basic components of a trauma system.[20] The details of the function and interrelationship of these components should be tailored to each trauma system's resources and needs. By defining the specifics of the components outlined below, the standards of care and thus the prospective components of QA are established (see Table 16-1).

Authority and Responsibility of Medical Direction (Table 16-2)

An integral part of any effective trauma system design is the designation of an agency with the responsibility and authority to manage and monitor the overall system. The role of oversight is most appropriately assumed by the agency that formally designates specific hospitals as trauma centers. The premise for this authority is that the process of designation carries with it the obligation to assure the public that the care delivered at a trauma center is of a higher level than that available at nondesignated hospitals or without a trauma system.[19]

To effectively perform this management responsibility the oversight agency, or EMSA, must have the authority to monitor the quality of care at all levels of the system and must have the power to effect necessary system alterations. The specifics of who selects the oversight agency, and what the scope of practice of this agency is in relation to trauma QA, should be defined as the trauma system is developed. This can be accomplished through state legislation, local consensus of involved parties, contractual agreements between the EMSA and the system participants, and/or the EMS policies and protocols. Since trauma systems may be viewed as a subset of the EMS system, the role of system overseer has been assigned to state, regional, or county EMS agencies in many states.[20]

The EMSA must design a QA program that includes monitoring of the *entire* trauma system to provide a meaningful evaluation of care of the injured patient.[20] The focus of trauma QA in the literature and often in practice has been on designated trauma-center care. Although it is important for trauma centers to perform in-hospital QA activities, it is equally important for the results of these activities to be integrated into a systemwide QA program. Both the trauma centers and the trauma system require collection and analysis of similar types of data, but the perspective and detail are different. Trauma center QA focuses on individual patients and individual practitioners. Trauma system QA evaluates *all* components of the system: system management, interactions between EMS agencies and/or EMS providers, quality of prehospital care, medical control, hospital care at designated trauma centers and at nondesignated hospitals, rehabilitation, and prevention.

EMS QA programs typically involve many of these components; what is unique about trauma system QA is the necessity of monitoring in-hospital care to determine if overall patient care is optimal. Rarely does an EMSA have a role in monitoring and evaluating the quality of in-hospital care, in providing feedback to the hospitals regarding such evaluation, and especially in recommending (or perhaps requiring) changes in individual or hospital practices.

Rather, the EMSA's authority over individual, hospital-based practitioners is limited to its relationship with the trauma center as a whole. The EMSA can discipline or decertify prehospital caregivers or dissolve contracts with EMS

Table 16-1. Prospective Components of a Trauma System

Components	Roles
A. Medical direction	
Authority	State legislation
	Local consensus
Responsibility	EMS contracts and policies
	Comprehensive system monitoring
B. Communications	
Dispatch centers	Specific trauma protocols
	Policies on response to trauma scenes
Base hospitals	Designation of specific trauma bases
	Base contact criteria
	Trauma logs
C. Training	
EMS agency	Role in education of trauma system members
	Specialized trauma training of EMS personnel
Prehospital providers	EMD training, BTLS, PHTLS
Trauma centers	ACS guidelines
	Trauma nurse core curriculum
	Outreach programs
Nondesignated facilities	Specialized trauma training of staff
	Trauma system policies and procedures
D. Triage	
Criteria	ACS guidelines
	Local variations

EMS, emergency medical services; EMD, emergency medical dispatch; BTLS, basic trauma life support; PHTLS, prehospital trauma life support; ACS, American College of Surgeons; BLS, basic life support; ALS, advanced life support; EMT-I, emergency medical technician-intermediate; EMT-P, emergency medical technician-paramedic.

providers; it cannot remediate or discipline hospital employees or physicians. The EMSA must rely on in-hospital QA committees, trauma directors, or hospital administrators to do this. The ultimate threat of discontinuing a trauma center's designation may be appropriate, but that threat may be an empty one if the trauma system would collapse without a specific trauma center (e.g., a county hospital). Hence, even if the authority of the EMSA over trauma systems is designated by law and even if the EMSA is the source of funding for trauma systems (such as through government grants), the ability of the EMSA to ensure that recommended changes are instituted is limited unless the relationship between EMS and the trauma centers is well defined (e.g., by contract), takes into consideration financial issues, and is characterized by a strong commitment by all parties to the goal of quality patient care.

Table 16-1. Prospective Components of a Trauma System—cont'd

Components	Roles
D. Triage (*continued*)	
In-hospital triage	Major trauma activation
	Minor trauma activation
Special considerations	Trauma center closure
E. Prehospital care	
Types of providers	First responders, BLS-EMT, ALS-EMT-I, EMT-P
Treatment protocols	Trauma scoring system
	Extent of field care
Times	Response
	Scene
	Transport
F. Transportation	
From field and interfacility	Level of personnel
	Ground versus air
	Guidelines and policies
G. Hospital care	
Level of designation	I, II, III, IV per ACS
Patient care	ACS guidelines and state or local requirements
Special considerations	Urban versus rural
H. Rehabilitation	
I. Prevention/Public Education	
EMS agency and trauma center	Injury prevention program
	Community education (including non-designated hospitals)
J. Medical evaluation (QA)	See text

Dispatch and Medical Control Hospital Communications

The dispatch center plays a pivotal role in the initial treatment of the trauma victim. Use of an emergency medical dispatch (EMD) program that includes specific trauma prearrival instructions and protocols ensures that necessary personnel arrive at the trauma scene in a safe and timely fashion. Coordination of dispatch activities with those of public-safety agencies is especially critical for trauma calls.

Medical control hospitals are those facilities designated by the EMSA to provide direct (or online) medical control to field personnel and to participate in prehospital QA and educational activities. In regions with more than one medical control hospital, designation of the medical control hospitals that are part of the trauma centers as specific "trauma bases" may be appropriate.

Table 16-2. Trauma System Components Necessary for Medical Direction

	Authority	Responsibilities	Personnel
EMS agency	Source—legislated by state Scope—state mandate	Designation of trauma centers based on ACS and/or local standards System management System QA	EMS medical director EMS administrator(s) Trauma coordinator(s) Data personnel
Trauma centers	Source—delegated by EMSA Scope—oversight of trauma care delivered in ED and inpatient settings	Patient care Participation in system and in-hospital QA Research ACS guidelines	Trauma director Trauma nurse coordinator Trauma registry personnel In-hospital QA personnel Administrator(s) ED medical director and nurse manager

ACS, American College of Surgeons; QA, quality assurance; EMSA, emergency medical services agency; ED, emergency department.

Training

Specific trauma training for all members of the trauma system is necessary to ensure high-quality trauma care. The American College of Surgeons (ACS) provides guidelines for training, such as Advanced Trauma Life Support (ATLS) and board eligibility for in-hospital personnel.[4] The level of training of all other system members, including EMS, emergency department and in-hospital staff of nondesignated hospitals, should be determined as the trauma system is being developed. As trauma systems age, personnel at nondesignated hospitals become less practiced at caring for the injured patient. However, as a result of undertriage by prehospital personnel or self-triage by patients, severely injured patients will occasionally arrive at nondesignated hospitals. Therefore emergency and surgical staff should maintain the skills necessary for initial stabilization of trauma victims (perhaps by way of courses) and be familiar with EMS trauma policies and interfacility transfer procedures.

The EMSA and trauma centers can optimize quality of trauma care by assisting in the development and implementation of training programs for all system members and by providing outreach programs to nondesignated hospitals and to the community.

Triage

The ACS has developed guidelines for field-trauma triage based on categorization of injury into three sets of criteria: 1) anatomic (e.g., penetrating trauma to the head, neck, or torso); 2) physiologic (e.g., revised trauma score [RTS]$\leq$3); and 3) mechanism of injury (e.g., vehicle rollover without restraints).[4] If a patient's injuries fit categories 1 or 2, transport to a trauma center is considered necessary. The third category is referred to as "paramedic judgment" in some systems; presence of these criteria suggests, but does not mandate, transport of the patient to a trauma center.[1] Although debate over the efficacy of these guidelines is ongoing, most systems use them in conjunction with variations based on local experience, resources, and political considerations.[2,18]

Field triage is not always accurate, and triage must be further evaluated on arrival to receiving facilities. Trauma-center closure, both permanent and temporary, complicates field triage and transport decisions and must be considered when triage protocols are developed.

Prehospital Care

Optimal prehospital trauma care is delivered when field providers are highly trained. A team of emergency medical technician–intermediate (EMT-I) trained first responders and paramedics (trained in BTLS or PHTLS) provides the highest level of care but may not be feasible in all systems, especially rural. Physician-directed development of straightforward prehospital treatment protocols and policies, based on current ACS standards and current EMS and trauma literature, is critical. This process includes selection of a trauma scoring system (e.g., RTS, CRAMS) and decisions regarding extent of field care (e.g., treat on-scene versus treat en route), criteria for medical control hospital contact, use of the pneumatic antishock trousers or other specialized equipment (e.g., splints and spinal immobilization devices), and mode of transport from the scene to the receiving facility (i.e., ground versus helicopter or fixed-wing aircraft). The impact of treatment protocols and policies on prehospital scene and transport times must be considered if the "golden hour of trauma" is to be maintained.

Interfacility Transportation

Interfacility transports of trauma patients must be conducted expeditiously, safely, and in accordance with state and federal regulations (Omnibus Budget Reconciliation Act/Consolidated Omnibus Reconciliation Act). The EMSA should develop specific policies that address the appropriate stabilization of patients prior to transfer, level of personnel (e.g., paramedic, registered nurse, physician, respiratory therapist) conducting the transfer, mode of transfer (ground versus air), and proper notification and documentation procedures. It is critical that specific mechanisms exist at transferring and receiving hospitals to ensure that inappropriate transfers or inappropriate refusals of transfers do not occur.

As previously discussed, education of all appropriate personnel at nondesignated hospitals and trauma centers regarding the EMS and trauma system and the interfacility transfer policies will prevent such mishaps.

Hospital Care

The ACS has developed extensive guidelines directed at providing optimal in-hospital care of the trauma patient.[4] For trauma centers these include standards on hospital organization, availability of specially trained personnel and hospital facilities (i.e., emergency departments, operating suites, and intensive care units), provision of specialized equipment (e.g., computed tomography [CT] scanners), and QA and education programs. Trauma centers are categorized as level I, II, III, or IV based on their ability to meet these standards.

The appropriate number and level of trauma centers to be designated in a given region should be chosen by considering factors such as geography, population density, maintenance of trauma-center personnel skills and experience, financial resources, and degree of commitment by the hospital and its personnel to the trauma system.[4] Tailoring the ACS guidelines to fit local resources may be necessary to develop the trauma system, but acceptance of such compromises initially may result in irreversible problems later. Subspecialty backup by neurosurgeons and orthopedic surgeons provides an example of this quandary. Lack of sufficient numbers of these surgeons interested in providing trauma-center coverage has prompted many systems in California to allow surgeons to provide backup at more than one trauma center simultaneously. Other trauma centers have offered fixed financial reimbursement for taking calls. Problems with timeliness of physician response, quality of patient care, and trauma center financial viability have resulted.

Rehabilitation

Trauma patients are often discharged from the trauma center to home with continuing homecare, to a rehabilitation center, or to a nondesignated hospital. Monitoring the care received by these patients provides more accurate outcome data and ensures continuation of high-quality care. If these resources are not available within the region, the EMSA and/or trauma centers should develop such programs or have prearranged transfer agreements with facilities in other regions.

Process

Concurrent Activities

The QA process components consist of the actual activities used to monitor the medical care delivered; this can be done concurrently or retrospectively.

Concurrent activities for the EMSA include site (trauma center) visits to view ongoing care, ride-alongs with prehospital personnel, and communication with dispatch to follow multicasualty incidents or to monitor hospital status (e.g., trauma center closures). Medical control hospitals are especially well positioned for concurrent auditing of prehospital trauma triage and treatment. Not only can they provide online medical direction for prehospital caregivers, but a base trauma log can be kept to track the destination of potential trauma patients and injured patients triaged to nondesignated hospitals. Paramedic ride-alongs by both medical control hospital and trauma center personnel are beneficial for evaluating paramedics and providing hospital-based caregivers with a perspective on the care of the patient from the moment of injury.

Concurrent activities at the trauma center include observation of house staff or staff physicians by the trauma director and observation of nurses caring for trauma patients by a trauma nurse coordinator.

Use of standard evaluation tools or forms can facilitate identification of either individual or institutional performance trends.

Retrospective Activities

For better or for worse, retrospective QA activities are the major focus of most trauma system evaluations. They are predicated on the existence of a (preferably) computer-based, systematic trauma registry[20] and an organized, preplanned method for review of the reports generated by the registry. The type of trauma registry and the method for review that the system selects are governed by cost and time considerations, but both are essential for effective QA.

The definition of a critical trauma patient (CTP), prospective, and a major trauma victim (MTV), retrospective, must be described before meaningful review can begin. It is essential that all participants in the system use common definitions and that, if possible, the system's definitions are similar to national standards.[20] Accurate definitions are important not only to appropriately monitor the system but also to determine resource needs based on the number of severely injured patients treated by the system.[3] Although many other terms are used, CTP is the term used to describe patients identified by prehospital triage protocols as requiring prompt evaluation by a trauma team capable of definitive intervention.[20] Usually these patients are triaged to a trauma center. There are as many variations of the definition of CTP as there are prehospital trauma-triage protocols. Prehospital identification of a CTP based on anatomic and physiologic factors is consistent among most systems; the variations exist within the mechanism of injury category.[2]

An MTV is a retrospectively derived identification of those patients who *should* have been treated at a trauma center. There are also multiple variations of this definition,[3] many of which are based on injury severity score (ISS) and/or abbreviated injury scale (AIS). The AIS was created to describe single traumatic injuries and is the foundation for methods used to assess *multiply* injured patients such as the ISS. The AIS is a list of several hundred injuries, each with an assigned severity score that can range from 1 (minor injury) to 6 (injury that is almost always fatal). To compute the ISS, injuries are also sorted into six body regions: 1) external, 2) head and neck, 3) thorax, 4) abdomen/pelvic contents, 5) spine, and 6) extremities. The highest AIS severity score for each of these six body regions is identified; the ISS is the sum of the squares of the three greatest AIS scores. ISS values range from 1 to 75; however, if a patient has any AIS score of 6, the ISS is automatically defined to be 75.[6]

For example, MTVs may be defined as being all patients with an AIS ≥ 3[1] or all patients with an ISS ≥ 15.[5] In a study at Johns Hopkins, a consensus panel defined an MTV by using a combination of AIS scores, age, and location of injury.[11] The ACEP suggests that MTVs be defined as being all patients admitted with certain hospital discharge diagnoses (ICD-9-CM diagnosis of 800.0 through 959.9) as a result of an acute traumatic event and one or more of the following: 1) transfer to or from another acute care facility (including patients transferred for evaluation but not admitted), 2) admission to an ICU, 3) hospitalization of 3 days or more, or 4) death.[20]

Baxt defines an MTV based on the resources required to treat an injured patient, characterized by the following: 1) any patient who requires a nonorthopedic operative procedure with positive findings within the first 48 hours of admission, 2) fluid resuscitation of more than 1 liter or transfusion to maintain a systolic blood pressure ≥ 90, or 3) invasive central nervous system monitoring with evidence of increased intracranial pressure and a positive CT scan.[3]

Once a CTP and MTV are defined the decisions regarding which cases should be audited can be made; based on the system's resources, it may be possible to review all CTPs or only feasible to review all MTVs or only all deaths. Other options include using audit filters (i.e., indicators) to identify specific cases that system members feel must be reviewed. A list of possible process and outcome indicators is included in the box on page 171.[5,20]

To perform any review, trauma cases (preferably all CTPs) should be entered into a trauma registry.

Trauma registry

SELECTION   A trauma registry is a comprehensive data base that quantifies the trauma system for its participants. The registry and the reports generated from it are probably the most important tools for effective retrospective QA. Because trauma registries can be expensive and labor intensive, careful selection using multiple criteria is critical.

System needs—Prior to reviewing various registries the trauma system participants should determine which characteristics of a trauma registry are important for the system itself and for its individual agencies or facilities. For example, will it only be used to generate simple standard reports, or will outcome trending and statistical analysis be required? Will the system participants want to use data from the registry for research, tracking trauma-specific costs, or other specific functions? Will the generation of ad hoc reports (i.e., those with variable subjects or formats) be necessary?

Indicators for Trauma System Audit

Process indicators

1. Prehospital
  a. System access—patient unattended at scene more than 8 minutes
  b. Triage protocols
    1) Adherence by field personnel
    2) Alterations made by medical control hospital personnel
    3) MTV triaged to nondesignated hospital
  c. Times
    1) Response time> _____ minutes (10)
    2) Scene time > _____ minutes (20)
    3) Transport time > _____ minutes (20)
  d. Treatment protocols
    1) Adherence by field or medical control hospital personnel
    2) Success/failure of field procedures
      a) Intubations
      b) Cricothyrotomies
      c) Pleural decompressions

2. Hospital—See Figure 16-3

3. Interfacility
  a. Patients transferred between hospitals
    1) From one trauma center to another trauma center
    2) From nondesignated facility to another nondesignated facility
    3) From nondesignated facility to a trauma center
  b. Patient admitted to nondesignated facility (not transferred)

4. Financial
  a. Overall cost of trauma care system
  b. Individual facility trauma-specific costs

Outcome indicators

1. Prehospital
  a. Patient inappropriately designated as major trauma victim (overtriage)
  b. Patient *not* designated as MTV (undertriage)

2. Hospital
  a. Readmits
  b. Deaths and complications
  c. Patient transferred to an inpatient rehabilitation facility
  d. Patient transferred to a skilled nursing or residential facility
  e. Patient treated at trauma center and released home in _____ days

3. Deaths
  a. Patient expired at the scene
  b. Patient expired at a nondesignated facility
  c. Patient expired at a trauma center
  d. Patient expired and not assigned a probability of survival value
  e. Patient expired and not autopsied

Cost— Not only must the initial hardware and software costs be identified, but most registries will incur maintenance and upgrade fees. Additionally, the costs of personnel time to perform data input, chart abstraction, report generation, and report review should also be considered. The agency responsible for these costs should be selected (e.g., county EMS agency, state EMS authority, participating trauma centers themselves). Cost effectiveness is an important consideration, but costs should not prevent any given trauma center's participation.

User friendliness— It is crucial, especially if funds for personnel are limited, that the registry be easy for the system participants to use. For example, if the registry requires knowledge of programming language to generate reports, the number of individuals who can use it may be limited.

Flexibility— The ability of the registry to be adapted to collect different data points as the trauma system evolves may be especially important for those interested in performing research or financial analysis. The more flexible the registry is intended to be, the more preplanning is necessary to identify and create new data sets.

Accuracy— Data input errors are inevitable. Programmed checks for critical data points aid consistency and accuracy.

Compatibility— The production of meaningful system reports is optimized when the trauma centers and EMSA use the same trauma registry. Although the details and extent of data entered and the reports generated may be different, compatibility of registries can expedite the audit process.

UTILIZATION

Reports— Once a registry is selected, system participants should decide what type of reports will be produced and which patients (e.g., all CTPs, all MTVs), categories and parameters of data (e.g., complications, time to operating room), and specific data sets will be entered into the registry.[5] To evaluate the entire trauma system, all sources of patients must be identified and considered for entry into the registry (see Figure 16-1).

CTPs are the patients identified by prehospital providers as being severely injured. Other injured patients, who are later identified as MTVs, may be incorrectly triaged (undertriaged) to nondesignated hospitals. Additionally, many seriously injured patients are brought by private (non-EMS) vehicle to both designated and nondesignated hospitals. Occasionally, a fatally injured patient is "missed," even with close monitoring of trauma patient flow; thus review of autopsies is essential.

Once these groups of patients are entered into the registry, it will identify and generate reports on individual patients meeting specific requirements set by the system participants (see Figure 16-2), which will then produce system reports (see Figure 16-3). For example, the registry can be programmed to identify all deaths and complications and all MTVs. Further audit indicators on MTVs may be selected, such as those shown in the box on page 171, to more specifically identify patients for physician or committee review and to produce data for analysis of trends.

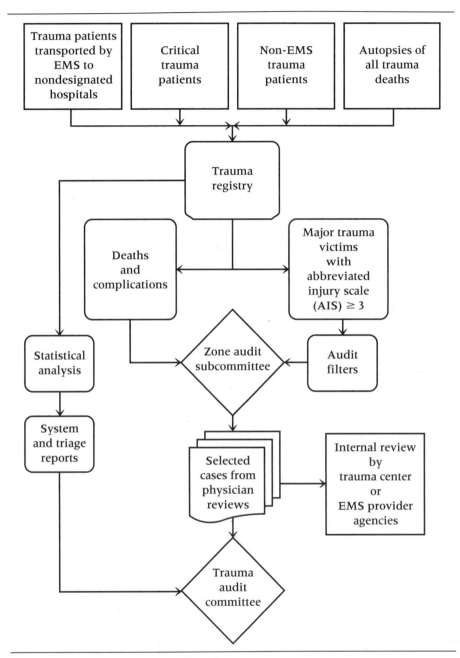

Figure 16-1 Process for review of individual patient care cases in a trauma system.

MTV with scene time > 20 min. .... yes	
Medical Record No.	: HI5344244
Age & Units	: 64 Y
Primary Tpt. Agency	: REG
Primary Mode of Tpt.	:
Triage Criterion	: H
Primary Env. of Injury	: AUTO FRONT PASSENGER
Primary Cause of Injury	: COLLISION WITH AUTO
GCS (Scene)	: 15
SBP (Scene)	: 240
RR (Scene)	: 20
Ped. TS (Scene)	: −7
GCS (Hosp)	: 15
SBP (Hosp)	: 180
RR (Hosp)	: 20
PEDPTS (Hosp)	: −7
Crystalloids (Trauma)	: 400
Packed Cells (Trauma)	:
Crystalloids (OR)	:
Packed Cells (OR)	:
ED Arrival Date	: 10/09/90
ED Arrival Time	:
ED Stay (Hours)	: 0.0
TRA Stay (Min)	: 30
Trauma Surgeon resp. (min)	: 0
Neurosurgeon resp. (min)	:
Anesthetist resp. (min)	: 50
OR Arrival Date	: 10/12/90
OR Proc. Start Time	: 0915 HR
ICU Stay (Days)	:
Injury Sev. Score	: 14
Prob. Surv. (RTS)	: 0.96
Hospital Length of Stay	: 16
Date of Discharge	: 10/25/90
Outcome	: Discharged Alive
OR Procedure Date	: 10/12/90
OR Procedure	: OPEN REDUCTION OF FRACTURE OF FEMUR W/INTERNAL FIXATION

Figure 16-2 Alameda County, California, patient summary report.
(Reprinted by permission of Alameda County Health Care Services.)

Readmit Proc. Date: No readmission procedures encountered

Injury Dx : B21.0 5 3
                FX OF SHAFT OR UNSPEC. PART OF FEMUR CLOSED
Injury Dx : 850.12 1 2
                850.12 1 2
Injury Dx : 910.0 6 1
                ABRASION OR FRICTION BURN OF FACE, NECK, & SCALP
                EXCEPT EYE. W/O INFECTION
Injury Dx : 873.31 6 1
                OPEN WOUND OF NASAL SEPTUM. COMPLICATED

No noninjury complications encountered
No Comments encountered

Figure 16-2 Continued

Indicators—Indicators are classified as system management, prehospital, hospital, or rehabilitation and further subdivided into process (i.e., delivery of care) or outcome (i.e., results of care).[20] Since the major purpose of system QA is to identify trends of care, the majority of system management indicators should focus on outcome evaluation, which will be discussed later in this chapter.

At a minimum, all deaths of seriously injured patients should be reviewed so that mortality rates can be determined and system problems identified (for example, if there is a high percentage of trauma deaths in the prehospital arena, further provider trauma education or an increase in the actual number of field personnel to better handle trauma victims might be indicated). Financial outcomes, such as cost of care at trauma centers or nondesignated hospitals, may also contribute information as to the efficiency of the trauma system. The impact of injury prevention programs on mortality and severity of injury may direct system management efforts.

Prehospital indicators should be selected according to resources available in the community, but such areas as system access, response times, efficacy of field triage and treatment protocols, and scene transport times provide vital information to EMS system managers.

One of the most important "outcomes" of a trauma system is properly matching the resources required to treat an injured patient with the injuries of that patient and, hence, appropriate triage to a designated trauma center for those patients most likely to benefit from the special capabilities of that center. It is also important to ensure that those patients who can adequately be cared for

System Report

Discharge Month: ___

I. Total trauma patients/Total major trauma victims

Highland	___/___
Eden	___/___
Children's	___/___
Total	___/___

II. Audit summary (referred to TAC)

	HGH (TAC)	EDEN (TAC)	CHMC (TAC)
Deaths	___	___	___
Complications	___	___	___
Readmits	___	___	___
Discharged from ED/Admitted	___	___	___
Lapsed time to OR > 2 hours	___	___	___
Unplanned return to OR in 24 hours	___	___	___
Epi/subdural not operated on	___	___	___
Age ≤ 14 admitted to adult center (CHMC ≥ 15)	___	___	___
Scene time > 20 min	___	___	___

III. Summary of deaths

	HGH	EDEN	CHMC
Died in ED	___	___	___
Died in OR	___	___	___
Died in ICU	___	___	___
Died on Ward	___	___	___

IV. Triss summary

	Patient	B/P	Hospital	ISS	Ps
Unexpected deaths		___	HGH		
		___	HGH		
Unexpected survivors		___	HGH		

Triage Report

Discharge Month: ___

I. Number of patients triaged

	Total	MTV	Blunt arrests
Highland	___	___	
Eden	___	___	
Children's	___	___	
Receiving hospitals	___	___	___
Overtriage rate ___		Undertriage rate ___	

II. Triage Criteria Summary (trauma centers only)

	Total	MTV
RTS ≤ 3	___	___
Penetrating injury to trunk/head	___	___
Two or more proximal long bone fractures	___	___
Traumatic amputation above wrist or ankle	___	___
Traumatic paralysis	___	___
Paramedic judgment	___	___
Death of other occupant	___	___
Extrication time > 20 minutes	___	___
Auto vs ped at ≥ 20 mph	___	___
Auto vs ped ≤ 14 or ≥ 55 years	___	___
Submersion with trauma	___	___
Significant blunt trauma to trunk/head	___	___
Vehicle rollover without restraints	___	___
MVA with high impact velocity	___	___
Falls ≥ 15 feet	___	___
Falls ≥ 10 feet, ages ≤ 14 or ≥ 55 years	___	___
Ejection of patient from vehicle	___	___
No criterion met	___	___
Unknown	___	___

V. *Z scores*

Penetrating   *Blunt*

VI. *Miscellaneous information*   *HGH*   *EDEN*   *CHMC*   *Total*

Nonactivations (total/MTV)

Organ donors

Patients to OR in 24 hours

VII. *Bypass report*

A: System   Total times ____   Total hours ____

B: Reason

CT   %____

  HGH

  EDEN

  CHMC

ED   %____

  HGH

  EDEN

  CHMC

OR   %____

  HGH

  EDEN

  CHMC

ICU   %____

  HGH

  EDEN

  CHMC

Other   %____

  HGH

  EDEN

  CHMC

C: Patient summary

Cause of injury   Hospital bypassed   MTV   Outcome

III. *Field procedures*	*Total*	*Blunt*	*Pen.*	*Lived*	*Died*
Intubated					
Cricothyrotomy					
MAST inflated					
Pleural decompression					

IV. *Helicopter transports* ____ ____

Destinations:

V. *Disposition of trauma center patients from ED*

	HGH	*EDEN*	*CHMC*	*%*
Admitted to ward				
Admitted to ICU				
Admitted to OR				
Discharged				
Transferred				
Died in ED				
Unknown				

Figure 16-3 Alameda County, California, trauma audit committee report. (Reprinted by permission of Alameda County Health Care Services Agency.)

at nondesignated hospitals are also correctly identified. By using process indicators (such as patient transfers from nondesignated hospitals to trauma centers and vice versa, deaths, complications, and length of hospitalization of MTVs inappropriately transported to nondesignated hospitals), the triage protocols can be appropriately revised to provide the maximum benefit to the maximum number of victims.

Hospital indicators should focus not only on outcomes such as death and complications but also on process factors such as MTVs' access to definitive care (e.g., time of arrival of trauma team and consultants and time to the operating room.)

It is important to regularly review the usefulness of all indicators selected for use in the trauma registry. Answers to such questions as "How often does a specific indicator identify cases that result in meaningful evaluation?"[7] may help refine the registry process.

General considerations—To maximize the usefulness of the trauma registry a specific agency or department should be assigned the responsibility for oversight at the system level and at each facility. Individuals within the agencies/facilities should be designated as responsible for coordination of the registry process. Additionally, a mechanism should exist to ensure patient confidentiality, such as the use of special access codes.[5,10] Therefore a commitment from all system members to participate in the registry is of the utmost importance and should be formalized by way of agreements or contracts between the EMSA and the trauma centers.

Audit committee

MEMBERSHIP AND PURPOSE The trauma registry produces data regarding individual patient care and trends in care and then performs statistical analysis on that data. It does not interpret the results or accomplish medical evaluation. A process that is time efficient, confidential, objective, and well planned must be delineated by each trauma system for this purpose. It is possible for one or two people at the EMSA or trauma centers to conduct review, but creation of a committee with representatives from the trauma system and the medical community maximizes objectivity. A sample membership for a Trauma Audit Committee (TAC) is shown in the box on page 179.

The major functions of the TAC are review of specified individual trauma patient cases; review of system and facility trends of care; determination of the appropriateness of trauma care; and recommendation as to necessary alterations of system, facility, or individual practices and policies.[1,19] Since responsibility for the overall medical care of the trauma victims rests with the EMSA, the committee should advise the EMS medical director. Additionally, if disagreement occurs among the members regarding committee decisions, it is best if the individual with a system perspective has the deciding vote.

REVIEW PROCESS The process for review of individual patient care cases is outlined in Figure 16-1 and described as follows:[1]

Sample Trauma Audit Committee Membership

Number of members	Type of members
1	EMS medical director (Chair)
1	EMS trauma coordinator
3	Trauma surgeon from each trauma-center hospital
3	Emergency department physician from each trauma-center hospital
1	Pediatric intensivist from pediatric trauma center
3	Representatives from local medical society (e.g., general surgeon, orthopedic surgeon, anesthesiologist, neurosurgeon)
1	Chief pathologist
1	EMS staff (alternates)
2	Physician representatives from nontrauma hospitals
Total members = 16	

Generation of individual patient registry reports— All MTVs selected by specified audit indicators and all deaths and complications are included in this group.

Review of reports at trauma centers— This may consist of detailed review and comment by the trauma director, review by the trauma nurse coordinator for accuracy of data input, or input to the report by in-hospital QA or mortality and morbidity committees. In general, such in-hospital reviews should *not* preclude further review of cases.

Review and triage of cases by pre-TAC subcommittee— In larger systems a pre-TAC process may be necessary to accomplish detailed review and select cases for further review by the TAC. Criteria should be set to determine which cases identified by the trauma-registry audit indicators merit further review and whether such cases should be referred back to the involved facility for further internal review and disposition or referred to the TAC. A classification system should be delineated for use at pre-TAC and TAC meetings. An example of such follows:[19]

Complications/Morbidity

1. Delay in diagnosis
2. Error in diagnosis
3. Error in judgment
4. Error in technique
5. Patient disease

Deaths

1. Probably preventable
2. Possibly preventable
3. Not preventable

Judgment of cases by the TAC—Cases are generally referred to the TAC when a decision regarding appropriateness of care (e.g., was death preventable) cannot be made definitively at the pre-TAC meeting or when a case is especially interesting or educational. The TAC also reviews and analyzes the system reports that include facility and system outcome measurements. Not only does this provide feedback to the system participants on the committee, it also allows the committee to identify trends and to make recommendations regarding modifications of facility or system processes.

Forwarding of committee (subcommittee and TAC) decisions and recommendations to EMS medical director—The duties of the audit committee end at this point. Further disposition of cases and system issues rests with the EMS medical director.

Other retrospective activities. The majority of retrospective auditing is accomplished through the trauma registry and the trauma committee review process. Other sources of retrospective evaluation that may be useful include: formal site (trauma center) surveys, performed either by the EMSA or by a consultant team; the EMS incident or unusual occurrence report system; and routine or focused audits performed at the trauma center, medical control hospital, or EMS provider agencies. Examples of focused audits that may be tracked and reported to the TAC and/or EMS medical director include: incidence of trauma center closure and/or bypass, summary of deaths, organ donations, success of field procedures, and patients going to the operating room within 24 hours of hospital admission.

Outcome

Statistical Analysis of Outcome Data

Statistical analysis of outcome data should be performed to focus retrospective audit processes; to produce objective evaluations of individual practitioner, facility, and system performance; and to compare these performances with national standards. The outcomes used for most analyses include deaths and complications and accuracy of field triage.

TRISS is a statistical methodology commonly used as the basis for measuring efficacy of trauma care.[6,7] It uses the trauma score (TS) or the RTS, both measures of physiologic severity of injury, and the ISS, a measure of anatomic severity of injury, to determine the probability of survival (Ps) of an individual patient. A patient with a Ps < 50% who survives is an "unexpected survivor." A patient with a Ps > 50% who dies is an "unexpected death." By calculating a Ps on all CTPs, the outliers (i.e., cases meriting further review) can be identified.

Additionally, by collating the Ps of all CTPs of a given trauma center or system and combining these with other parameters such as number of observed survivors and size of study population, the Z score can be calculated. The Z score is a means of assessing the statistical significance between the observed (A) and expected (E) survival rates following trauma. It provides an objective measure of an institution's or individual practitioner's patient survival rate as compared with norms developed by the Major Trauma Outcome Study (MTOS).

Terms such as *expected rates, norms,* or *standard values* refer to data obtained from the MTOS. These norms were derived using data from confirmed consecutive patients at 51 institutions (15,754 patients with blunt injuries and 7,423 with penetrating injuries). Regression rates or coefficients were determined from these data and are used in standardized formulas to calculate Z, W, M, and other statistical scores. The coefficients and formulas can be incorporated into a trauma registry (commercial registry software packages provide this capability) and allow routine computations of trauma center and/or system data.[6]

There are some limitations to the "power" of the Z (i.e., its probability of detecting a specific difference between A and E as being significant).[8] Variables such as sample size, magnitude of the difference, definition of CTP, and distribution of the Ps in the study population can all influence the accuracy of the Z score. Therefore the W score was developed to describe the clinical and practical significance of the differences between A and E. The W score represents the average increase or decrease in the number of survivors per 100 patients treated compared with the norm as defined by the MTOS. M, another statistical measurement, describes how accurate the match is between a given patient population and the patient population that provided the MTOS data.

The overtriage rate (OTR) and undertriage rate (UTR) are also outcome measurements for the trauma system since they measure efficacy of care delivered.[20] To obtain true rates the denominator must include *all* patients triaged by the EMS system (i.e., all CTPs) regardless of whether they are transported to trauma centers or to nondesignated hospitals. Thus the definition of a CTP can markedly influence calculations.

$$OTR = \frac{\text{number of non-MTVs transported to trauma center}}{\text{total number of patients triaged by EMS}}$$

$$UTR = \frac{\text{number of MTVs transported to nondesignated hospitals}}{\text{total number of patients triaged by EMS}}$$

It is essential that the OTR and UTR be consistent in their definition and application within and between systems. Comparing these rates before and after alterations in system design can indicate the success of such changes. As triage protocols are made more restrictive in an attempt to decrease the OTRs, more patients who are seriously injured (and later identified as MTVs) are transported to nondesignated hospitals (i.e., the UTR increases). If triage protocols are less restrictive in their definition of CTPs, more patients will be transported to the trauma center who may not truly need such specialized services. Clearly, both patient care and costs of care are impacted when the UTR and OTR increase.

Current studies indicate that a UTR of less than 5% is most appropriate. OTRs studied are highly variable, but the average rate appears to be approximately 40%.[2]

Other rates that may be useful for system outcome measurement include mortality rates (i.e., preventable, nonpreventable, probably preventable) and complication rates. If the trauma system allows trauma center closure and bypass, bypass rates of each trauma center are also important.

Identification of Outcome Trends

By collating data obtained from concurrent and retrospective audit activities and statistical analysis of outcome data, outcome trends for all components of the trauma system can be identified. Table 16-3 summarizes the sources and results of outcome evaluations.

Feedback

Once outcome trends are identified, the process of closure of the feedback loop may be accomplished. The benefits of an effective QA system are often realized at this point. Data provided by analysis of trauma registry reports and statistical derivations provide objective support for EMS recommendations. The steps necessary to attain this goal include: 1) communication of results of QA activities (i.e., outcome trends) to appropriate system participants; 2) investigation to identify reasons for deviations from norm; 3) recommendations for modifications necessary to return performance to norm; 4) institution of modifications; and 5) reevaluation of performance (see Figure 16-4).

The process for accomplishing closure of the feedback loop must also be well defined and ensure maintenance of patient and provider confidentiality. Specific steps for handling identified problems with individual, agency, or system performance are as follows:

Individual performance
1. Referral of EMSA's findings and recommendations to internal QA system
   a. Prehospital—QA section of provider agency
   b. Hospital—QA committee, trauma committee, or departmental committees
2. Commendation, counseling, reeducation, remediation, or discipline of individual according to agency's/hospital's standard procedures
3. Report of disposition of case back to EMSA
4. Changes in provider agency, hospital, and/or EMS policies and procedures, if appropriate

Provider agency or hospital performance
1. Reports at audit committee
2. Referral of specific concerns by EMSA to provider agency or hospital administration and/or trauma service

Table 16-3. Outcome Trends

System component	Source of evaluation	Outcome results
Prehospital	Statistical comparison between CTPs and MTVS	OTR
		UTR
	Ride-alongs	Individual provider performance
	Retrospective PCR audits	
	TAC review of cases	Provider agency performance (dispatch, BLS, ALS)
	OTRs, UTRs	
	EMS site visits	Medical control hospital performance
	Base hospital or EMS review of prehospital run reports and tapes	
	OTRs, UTRs	
Hospital	Z and W scores	Physician performance compared with established norm
	Mortality and complication rates	
		Hospital performance compared with established norm
Overall system	System Z and W scores	System performance compared with established norm
	System mortality and complication rates	
	Change in rates of preventable deaths	Impact of system
	Mortality and disability rates	
	Trauma-specific costs at nondesignated and designated hospitals and for prehospital care— provider agencies and EMSA	Cost of trauma system

CTP, critical trauma patient; MTV, major trauma victim; OTR, overtriage rate; UTR, undertriage rate; PCR, prospective, randomized, controlled; TAC, trauma audit committee; BLS, basic life support; ALS, advanced life support; EMSA, emergency medical services agency.

3. Changes in agency, hospital, departmental policies and procedures, or alteration of contract with EMS as appropriate
4. Education programs to address issues identified by trend analysis
5. EMS site surveys to ensure capability of trauma center to effect changes and to audit compliance with changes

System performance
1. Report at audit committee
2. Referral to appropriate EMSA section or committee
3. Alterations of EMS policies, protocols, or procedures, as appropriate

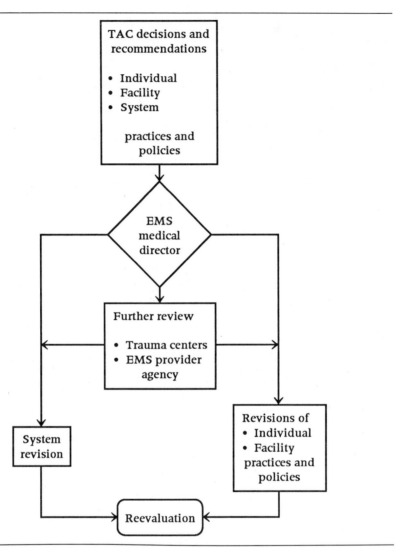

Figure 16-4 Closure of audit feedback loop.

4. Changes in design of system (designation of trauma centers, medical control hospitals, providers, etc.) as appropriate
5. Educational programs
6. Dissemination of changes in system protocols, design, etc.
   a. Trauma audit or medical review committees
   b. Newsletters

A critical component of the feedback process that ensures closure of the feedback loop is reevaluation. Once alterations in the trauma system's structure or process components are made, it is essential that compliance by individuals and agencies be monitored and that the effect on outcome measurements be determined. For example, if the QA process determines that the trauma-triage protocols result in the transport of too many severely injured patients to nondesignated hospitals (perhaps reflected by a high number of trauma deaths at these facilities and a high UTR), the EMS medical director may decide to broaden the definition of a CTP. This will require revisions of protocols (structure), education of field providers regarding the new protocols, monitoring of provider adherence to the new protocols, and recalculation of the UTR and the OTR. It also may require analysis of the financial impact of sending more injured patients to the trauma center. The EMS medical director, with input from the system participants, must then use this information to reevaluate the system's performance and to develop the solution that best meets the overall needs and goals of the system.

Financial Considerations

It is clear from the available literature—both scientific and popular—that the cost of trauma systems is a topic of much controversy.[3] The purpose of regionalization of trauma care is to improve the quality of care delivered to injured patients. Since it costs money to care for patients regardless of where they receive the care, it does not seem inherently obvious that the cost would be greater by centralizing care. In fact, limiting the number of hospitals that must provide readily available specialized care and services might actually decrease the total cost of caring for injured patients.

The creation of a trauma system, however, usually does result in an absolute increase in the level of service offered in a region and, therefore, in additional expenses for the system members. The total cost of the trauma system includes: trauma-specific costs at designated hospitals; specialized education, training, personnel, and equipment costs for prehospital providers and for EMS agencies; education costs for nondesignated hospitals; and costs for trauma QA.

Trauma centers have discovered that their costs have increased mostly as a result of the high cost of upgrading resources (both human and equipment) to obtain trauma center designation. Indeed, the cost of treating a trauma victim is 2 times greater than that of a cancer patient and 3 times that for a cardiovascular patient.[22] Additionally, it is difficult to prospectively identify a patient who truly needs the specialized care at trauma centers; therefore the creation of a trauma system may result in an increase in the number of patients receiving (perhaps unnecessarily) such high-cost care. Simultaneously, factors such as poor payer mix, limitation of reimbursement by third-party payers, and increasing numbers of indigent trauma victims have resulted in decreased revenues for trauma centers and EMS provider agencies.

There are, however, sources of funding available for trauma centers and systems. In some counties, tax assessments for trauma care or EMS systems direct monies from the taxpayer to the trauma oversight (usually EMSA) agency. Such funds may be used to educate prehospital caregivers, subsidize trauma centers, or reimburse the EMSA for QA activities. State or federal EMS grants or trauma care grants are also a source of funding.[17] The Trauma Care Systems Planning and Development Act of 1990 (HR 1602) may also provide such aid.[21] Some trauma systems have trauma centers that make a profit and pay a fee to the EMSA for trauma center designation. Although not always a source for trauma care itself, such monies may be used to support QA activities.[19]

Even if a trauma center or system is able to collect in revenues what it expends or can obtain a stable funding source, the overall cost of trauma care to society may be greater with these systems than without them. Trauma victims comprise a relatively small proportion (less than 2%) of emergency patients. However, they are usually younger than the general patient population, so that saving a life or decreasing disability may result in the retrieval of more potentially productive years of life.

Do these benefits, however, justify the high cost? The future of trauma care is at least partly dependent on the answer to this question. This answer will be provided by 1) accurately assessing and analyzing the financial impact of the overall trauma system, including costs of the system and its impact on direct and indirect costs of decreased morbidity and mortality; and 2) objectively supporting the premise that a given trauma system delivers a higher quality of care than that available without such a system.

Both of these tasks can be accomplished by an effective trauma QA program. Of course, the QA process itself costs money. A study[19] involving the San Diego County trauma system reported an annual cost of approximately $300,000 for detailed QA review of severely injured patients. Alameda County (also in California) spends approximately $250,000 annually for the personnel and equipment necessary to conduct the entire trauma QA program. However, it should be noted that Alameda County's EMS district (a tax-assessment district) provides more than $5 million annually to subsidize local trauma centers and that this subsidy is less than 25% of the overall cost of the trauma system. Thus a trauma QA program that not only focuses its efforts on the structure, process, outcome, and feedback components of QA but also uses data derived from these activities to address the financial aspects of trauma care is itself cost effective. Allocation of resources based on objective data ensures that the goal of low-cost/high-benefit care will be attained.

Summary

The preceding sections have presented an ideal trauma QA plan that is a combination of many systems' plans, most of them large urban/suburban counties or regions. The basic QA components discussed are necessary for any effective QA plan but can be tailored to the local financial resources and political environment. What is most important is that the QA program be well planned and well defined and that it accomplishes, by constant evaluation, modification, and reevaluation, the goal of high-quality care at a reasonable cost to the benefit of the most people.

REFERENCES

1. Alameda County Health Care Services Agency: *Alameda County EMS policy manual,* 1991, The Agency.
2. Baxt WG, Jones G, Fortlage D: The trauma triage rule: a new, resource-based approach to the prehospital identification of major trauma victims, *Ann Emerg Med* 19:1401-1406, 1990.
3. Baxt WG, Upenieks V: The lack of full correlation between the injury severity score and the resource needs of injured patients, *Ann Emerg Med* 19:1396-1400, 1990.
4. Caring for the injured patient, *Bull Am Coll Surgeons,* 71(10): Oct 1986.
5. Cales RH et al: Trauma registries, *Trauma Quarterly* 5(3):1-8, 1989.
6. Champion HR, et al: The Major Trauma Outcome Study: establishing national norms for trauma care, *J Trauma* 1356-1365, 1990.
7. Committee on Injury Scaling: *Abbreviated Injury Scale 1985 revision,* Arlington Heights, Ill, 1985, American Association for Automotive Medicine.
8. Cottington EM, Shufflebarger CM, Townsend R: The power of the statistic: implications for trauma research and quality assurance review, *J Trauma* 1500-1509, 1989.
9. Eastman AB et al: Regional trauma system design: critical concepts, *Am J Surg* 79-87, 1987.
10. Gillot AR, Thomas JM, Forrester C: Development of a statewide trauma registry *J Trauma* 1667-1672, 1989.
11. MacKenzie EJ, Steinwachs DM, Ramzy AI: evaluating performance of statewide regionalized systems of trauma care, *J Trauma* 30(6):681-687, 1990.
12. Maull KI et al: Trauma center verification, *J Trauma* 521-524, 1986.
13. Pollack DA, McLain PW: Trauma registries, *JAMA* 2280-2283), 1989.
14. Pories SE et al: Practical evaluation of trauma deaths, *J Trauma* 1607-1610, 1989.
15. Report from the 1988 Trauma Registry Workshop, including recommendations for hospital-based trauma registries, *J Trauma* 827-834, 1989.
16. Sacco WJ et al: Partition: a quantitative method for evaluating prehospital services for trauma patients, *Comp Biol Med,* 221-227, 1988.
17. Scheib BT, Thompson ME, Kerns TJ: Federal influences on the development of trauma registries, *J Trauma,* 835-841, 1989.
18. Selden BS, Schnitzer PG, Nolan FX: Medicolegal documentation of prehospital triage, *Ann Emerg Med* 19(5):547-551, 1990.
19. Shackford SR, Hollinsworth-Fridlund P, McArdle and Eastman AB: Assuring quality in a trauma system—the medical audit committee: composition, cost and results, *J Trauma* 866-875, 1987.
20. *System Audit Appendix to Trauma System Guidelines for Trauma Care System.* In: *Trauma Care Systems Quality Assurance Guidelines,* 1990, American College of Emergency Physicians.
21. *Trauma Care Systems Planning and Development Act of 1990,*
22. Yoon D: Trauma care: future shock, *CAL/ACEP Lifeline,* 1991.

Section Four

Special Roles in Quality Management

EMS systems across the country have used a variety of innovative methods, implemented by distinct individuals, to improve care in their areas. The intense scrutiny and beneficial effects brought to an EMS system by research and field review of care are presented in this section. The important contributions and potential assistance that may be gleaned from the state lead agency are also identified. Finally, the role of the paramedic coordinator, who serves as the linchpin of quality efforts in many systems, is addressed.

17

State EMS Offices in the Quality Assurance Process

Barak Wolff, M.P.H.
Timothy Fleming, M.D.

This chapter specifically addresses the roles, responsibilities, and opportunities for state-level emergency medical services (EMS) lead agencies to participate in and to affect the quality assurance (QA) process to ensure that the public is served in an appropriate, accessible, consistent, and medically accountable manner. Similarities and differences in state-level organization, funding, function, and attitude are summarized. The critical relationship between the state lead agency and local EMS systems to ensure quality care is also discussed.

EMS as a structured component of both the health-care delivery system and the public safety/emergency response system is less than 25 years old. Prior to the late 1960s, EMS simply did not exist as an organized, recognized, or even conceptualized public service. The rapid development of EMS in the United States over the past several decades has been stimulated by events, personalities, leadership, funding initiatives, and rising public expectations at all levels—local, statewide, and national.

The late 1970s and the 1980s saw the legal definition, description, and regulation of EMS by each of the states and territories. In each state a state lead agency for EMS now exists that has some role to play in ensuring the quality of care. However, in most cases the actual operation and delivery of EMS rests with local areas, either as a direct function of city or county government or as a partnership between private and public entities. The federal contribution has consisted primarily of conceptualizing EMS system functioning, providing funds to state and regional organizations for EMS planning and implementation, developing national standard training curricula and consensus standards, and supporting EMS-related research.

Overview of State EMS Lead Agencies

This section briefly describes the overall organization and function of state-level EMS lead agencies. It draws heavily on two resources: the *Standard Guide for Structures and Responsibilities of EMS Systems Organizations,* as developed by the American Society for Testing and Materials Committee F-30, and the 1988 and 1991 monographs, *The EMS Office: Its Structure and Functions,* produced by the National Association of State EMS Directors.[1,3] The former is a conceptualization of what "ought to be," whereas the latter is a description of what was in place in the late 1980s. A third recommended resource is a chapter, "State and Regional EMS Systems," taken from the *Principles of EMS Systems.*[2]

Because the public has a right to expect a certain minimum quality of health service and care, generally state governments define and guarantee that minimum. Accordingly, the vast majority of states have passed legislation providing formal structure to EMS, recognizing it as a vital public service that must be planned, coordinated, supported, evaluated, monitored, and regulated to ensure that those minimum expectations are met. This basic rationale for state involvement in EMS parallels that of laws governing occupational licensing, certification and licensing of health-care facilities, regulation of motor carriers, etc., all of which have been around for many decades. States, however, are not the only level of government that has a legitimate interest in EMS. Some local jurisdictions may enact their own standards that are broader and more stringent than that of the state. In some cases there is an overriding national interest that allows the federal government to establish standards, as in the case of interstate commerce.

Location of and Direction to State EMS Offices

In most states EMS legislation identifies a lead agency that is charged with a variety of responsibilities and empowered with the authority to carry out certain regulatory functions. First and foremost EMS is concerned with the delivery of medical care; therefore, most states have placed the lead-agency responsibilities within the state health agency. Exceptions to this include independent EMS commissions (e.g., Kansas and Maine), Department of Education (e.g., Ohio), Department of Human Resources (e.g., District of Columbia), Emergency Management Agency (e.g., Indiana), university-based (e.g., Maryland), hospital-based (e.g., Virgin Islands), or separate state agency (e.g., American Samoa and California). In all other states the EMS lead agency is located within the state health agency. About 80% of the EMS offices were created and mandated by legislation, whereas the remaining 20% were created administratively or by executive order.

In all but a handful of states the EMS lead agency has some type of advisory council to guide or, in some cases, direct the lead agency. Most state-level EMS advisory councils are mandated by legislation and are appointed by the governor or the secretary of the health department. Although their specific composition varies, these councils generally include multidisciplinary representation from groups such as prehospital EMS providers, EMS agencies, nurses, physicians, hospital administrators, fire service members, law enforcement, EMS educators, and the public. Each of these "stakeholders" has the opportunity to play a role in the planning, development, and implementation of the EMS system. Most state EMS councils provide advice on policy direction and priority setting and frequently act as EMS advocates. Perhaps most importantly, these councils can serve as a forum for the cooperative action that is required for optimal EMS system functioning.

State Funding

Funding support for the lead agency varies considerably from less than $300,000 per year for some states to more than $10,000,000 per year in several others (which include funds that are passed through in support of local EMS provider organizations). In 1987 approximately $54 million was provided to state EMS lead agencies by state general funds, approximately $16 million by the federal Preventive Health Block Grant, approximately $4 million by Section 402 National Highway Traffic Safety Administration (NHTSA) funds, and $7 million by other sources. In addition, special or dedicated EMS funds in about 13 states provided more than $50 million in additional revenue, the majority of which went to support local EMS agencies through grants and contracts. In 1987 the annual per capita state funding for EMS ranged from less than $.10 in Wisconsin, Oklahoma, and Iowa to more than $10 in Hawaii and Maryland.

Roles and Responsibilities

The enormous range in state expenditures for EMS is indicative of the wide variation in roles and responsibilities that are undertaken by state EMS offices. As reflected in Table 17-1, the core EMS office functions accomplished by almost all states, either directly by the state EMS office or by another agency, involve the training standards, testing, licensing (certification) and regulation of prehospital personnel, and regulation of ground ambulance services. (Some states *license*, whereas others *certify* their emergency medical technicians [EMTs]. This chapter uses license as the generic term.) In addition, the development of a statewide EMS plan and an EMS communication plan is a common function. Both of these should be accomplished with considerable input and review from local EMS participants to ensure an accurate reflection of the current reality and shared future vision. These are often accomplished under the guidance and auspices of the state-level EMS advisory council. Responsibilities such as facility categorization and/or designation, protocol development, air ambulance regulation, coordination of disaster response, and others further down the list are either secondary functions, accomplished by another agency, or are not undertaken at all.

Table 17-1. Functions of State EMS Offices

In the following table the first column shows duties that might reasonably be performed in an EMS system. The second column is a count of those states in which the EMS office is primarily responsible for the function; the third, a count of states in which some other state agency is primarily responsible; the fourth, a count of states in which the EMS office has secondary responsibility for the function (typically, states in which some other agency has primary responsibility); and the fifth, a count of states in which the function is not performed. EMS regions count as "other agencies" within this table. The functions most often performed by EMS offices are presented first.

	Function performed by what agency?			
Function	EMS office	Another	EMS secondarily	None
Adopt basic written test	36	7	3	0
License basic personnel	36	7	2	1
Adopt basic practical test	35	7	3	1
Regulate basic personnel	35	7	4	2
Establish EMS plan	33	10	4	1
Administer advanced written test	31	14	2	0
Adopt basic curricula	31	10	6	1
License ambulance services	31	11	1	2
Regulate ground services	31	12	7	0
Adopt advanced written test	30	13	5	0
Inspect ground vehicles	30	14	2	1
License advanced personnel	30	13	4	1
Administer basic written test	29	16	6	0
Regulate advanced personnel	29	13	8	2
Adopt advanced curricula	28	14	7	0
Adopt statewide advanced test	28	13	5	3
Approve each ALS course	28	11	3	2
Approve individual BLS courses	28	12	4	1
Establish EMS communications plan	28	13	5	4
Certify instructors	25	12	3	6

ALS, advanced life support; BLS, basic life support; DNR, do not resuscitate; CE, continuing education; ED, emergency department.
National Association of State EMS Directors: *The emergency medical services offices: structure and function,* Council of State Governments, Lexington, Ky, 1991.

Personnel and Service Regulation

In considering the role of the state EMS office in the QA process, it is through the regulation of prehospital personnel and services that both the "scope of practice" and the "standard of care" receive their initial definition. In approving training programs and administering the written and practical examinations for licensure

Table 17-1. Functions of State EMS Offices—cont'd

Function	Function performed by what agency?			
	EMS office	Another	EMS secondarily	None
Inspect air vehicles	25	11	1	8
Regulate air services	24	11	6	7
License air ambulance services	23	10	2	11
Set vehicle standards	23	18	6	1
Establish EMS regions & councils	22	15	2	4
Administer basic practical test	21	27	6	0
Coordinate EMS disaster response	21	22	7	2
Administer advanced practical test	19	24	3	2
Deliver instructor training	18	20	10	4
Categorize trauma centers	15	20	2	10
Designate trauma centers	14	19	2	11
Establish treatment protocols	14	30	5	1
Establish transfer protocols	13	30	2	3
Establish triage protocols	13	29	4	2
Categorize other spec. centers	7	22	3	15
Establish DNR protocols	7	31	2	9
Hire regional EMS staff	7	22	1	13
Set regional EMS policy	7	24	4	11
Deliver basic training	6	41	6	0
Certification of need for ambulances	4	21	5	21
Deliver advanced training	4	42	4	1
Designate other specialty centers	4	20	0	21
Operate training academy	3	27	3	17
Regulate ambulance rates	3	19	1	25
Approve training centers	1	0	0	0
Approve CE training centers	1	0	0	0
Inspect hospital EDs	1	32	3	8
License emergi-care center	0	22	0	20

at the various prehospital levels, the state EMS office delineates the minimally acceptable training and performance criteria for basic providers.

Over the past 15 years most states have adopted the EMT-basic level, the national standard curriculum published by the U.S. Department of Transportation (DOT), which has resulted in highly uniform performance expectations among different states. This is less true at the EMT-paramedic level and not at all true for EMT-intermediates. Some states take the responsibility for defining the local scope of practice more formally and actually develop and issue mandatory statewide protocols that spell out exactly what field personnel can and cannot do. The majority of states, however, provide sample protocols that are in keeping with the licensure regulations, which local services are encouraged to adapt to local needs.

States define not only the substance or content of knowledge and skills that leads to licensure of EMTs, but also the process for obtaining and maintaining licensure, generally through regulations. This is another part of the state's effort to ensure quality and protect the citizenry. In addition to course completion and successful examination, many states require additional certifications such as cardiopulmonary resuscitation, advanced cardiac life support, and prehospital trauma life support. States may also require applicants to disclose any criminal convictions that might influence the decision to grant licensure. Some states require evidence of affiliation with a service provider, whereas others require a physician medical director's sign-off evidencing support and competency, particularly at the advanced life support (ALS) levels.

Licensure renewal is another aspect of this state-level QA effort. Although requirements vary considerably, EMTs generally must present evidence of continuing education and/or formal refresher training, often in addition to current certifications and support from the medical director. However, there is great disparity among states regarding the frequency and requirements for EMT licensure renewal. In 1987 several states (e.g., Kansas, Delaware, and Georgia) required annual licensure renewal. The majority of states are split between two- and three-year renewal periods, and several (e.g., Texas and Virginia) allow for a four-year renewal. States are also split closely on whether a formal written and practical exam is required for licensure renewal. From the state perspective, the requirement for a medical director's sign-off or endorsement is generally verified simply by a signed statement. However, at the service or system level this affords an opportunity to tie this required support to demonstrated competency in keeping with the local QA plan.

In regulating EMS provider agencies the primary consideration is again the protection of the public through QA. In most cases, states develop regulations that set forth minimum expectations for organizational integrity (capitalization, insurance, bonding, etc.), staffing, vehicles, equipment, communications capability, operational characteristics, medical direction, and even local QA. Such regulations may mandate the use of a prehospital medical record or documentation of periodic case reviews supervised by the service's medical director. For example, about 75% of the states require that ALS providers have a medical director, whereas only 25% of states require a medical director at the basic life support (BLS) level.

The ability of the EMS community to influence such regulations through active participation in the developmental process can have a major impact on the level and quality of care provided throughout the state, as well as the minimum QA activities expected within each service. That a service has met these expectations must be demonstrated in the initial application and through subsequent periodic inspections and complaint investigations. These minimum expectations then become the standards of care for ambulance operations in that state. The capacity and will of the state EMS office to actually enforce these standards varies considerably, particularly if the inspections are accomplished by another agency.

The same is true for the regulations governing the training, licensing, and licensure renewal for field personnel and for other aspects of the EMS system, such as trauma systems development, distribution of grants funds, etc. The development of regulations through law and practice needs to be a very public and participatory process. Drafts should be widely circulated for review and comment. In addition to formal public hearings, informal community meetings should be offered to discuss new regulations, receive feedback, and answer questions. Ultimately, regulations are most effective when they reflect a strong consensus of opinion.

Other Functions

State EMS offices may provide a wide variety of other functions, including planning and coordination, technical assistance, funding support, data collection and evaluation, professional liaison, public education and information, prevention and injury control programs, disaster preparedness and response planning, systems development and monitoring (including the designation of critical care facilities), specialty training, and much more. Many of these functions can have some relationship, either direct or indirect, to QA efforts.

For example, many state EMS offices, either directly or in conjunction with regional EMS offices, are available to provide technical assistance to local communities about all aspects of their EMS system. This can include an evaluation of local system performance, an assessment of the various EMS components, and/or recommendations for system improvement. It is often through such technical assistance that the state can influence the upgrading of training, the increased funding for medical direction, the creation of a local EMS advisory board, and the like. The state can provide sample material, such as medical director contracts, run forms, QA plans, continuing education programs, and disaster plans, that both help alleviate the need for each local area to "rediscover the wheel" and promote consistency among jurisdictions.

In difficult policy areas, such as living wills, do not resuscitate (DNR) orders, drug testing, and initiating/stopping resuscitation, the state office can play a range of productive roles from actually promulgating a statewide policy to developing sample policies for local consideration to providing appropriate information and technical assistance. These issues can be very difficult, confusing, and sensitive and can cause major medical-legal problems for local areas to deal with. The state office can be of enormous assistance in providing guidance in these areas of evolving importance.

As in any health-care delivery setting, the medical record is essential not only for medical-legal documentation but also as the basis for QA activities. About half the states either mandate or offer a prehospital medical record or run form for local use. From these forms, many states not only provide summary data to local services but also have the ability to aggregate information on both a regional and statewide basis to stimulate QA discussions. For example, if a review of all serious trauma runs reveals that only 60% are receiving oxygen therapy, there is clearly a problem with reporting, performance, and/or training that needs to be addressed. Even at a statewide level, such simple analyses can raise important questions and become a basis of comparison for local system evaluation. Whether provided by the state or not, an effective run form and/or data collection system is essential for QA. Two concerns often expressed about statewide systems is that they are an expensive undertaking for a state office, which may detract from other functions, and they often do not provide adequate information and feedback to larger and more urban services whose information needs may be extensive.

Another function of the state EMS office may be to request and coordinate an assessment of the state EMS system by the NHTSA. To accomplish this, the NHTSA assembles a group of experts with demonstrated leadership and expertise though involvement in national EMS organizations. This technical assistance team (TAT) assembles at an agreed-upon location (usually the state capital) and listens to in-depth briefings from the state EMS staff. Topics typically addressed include resource management, regulation and policy, manpower and training, transportation, facilities, communication, evaluation, public information and education, and medical direction and/or control. Special issues can also be covered as required by the specific state. The TAT then prepares a response addressing the standard in the area, the status within the state, and recommendations to improve the particular section. The state may then use these recommendations to revise EMS policy, structure, funding, etc., as they see fit.

Medical Direction

The majority of states have a full- or part-time position for a state EMS medical director. In a 1988 survey conducted by the NASEMSD, of 46 states and territories responding, 31 reported having an EMS medical director. Of these, 17 were part-time contracted positions, 6 were appointed, and 6 were state employees. In most cases the state medical director reports to the state EMS director.

The primary function of the state medical director is to provide overall medical direction for the statewide system and to ensure the medical appropriateness of state regulations and policies. Although the position is technically advisory in nature, the responsibilities are genuine and the opportunity for influence is great. State EMS medical directors must maintain productive relationships with the broader medical community and provide technical assistance and support to local EMS medical directors. In many states EMS physician forums have been formed to foster information sharing, continuing education, creative problem solving, and networking. For physicians at the local level who are new to the roles and responsibilities of being an EMS medical director, this technical assistance and support from a knowledgeable state-designated physician has proven to be invaluable.

It is essential that state EMS medical directors be licensed physicians with formal training in emergency medicine and experience in both online and offline EMS medical control. They should have good written and verbal communication skills and be actively involved with various emergency medicine professional groups. Most importantly, state EMS medical directors must be accessible to provide the necessary support and advice to maximize the potential of this position.

Characteristics of Sound Lead EMS Agency Functioning

States vary considerably in their priorities and basic attitude toward their lead agency responsibilities, which range from technical assistance and/or support (participatory) to regulatory (control). Although all state EMS offices perform elements of both roles, their relative priority is primarily a function of the state's overall political climate and secondarily a product of history and leadership styles. For example, in states in which strong government control is uncommon, state EMS offices are more likely to be heavily involved in the provision of technical assistance and support, and vice versa. In general, the most effective and respected state EMS offices tend to balance these responsibilities; they are by no means mutually exclusive.

Of critical importance to the effective functioning of the state EMS office is the facilitation and encouragement of broad participation in the process of developing regulations. EMS is an extremely dynamic environment subject to rapid changes driven by professional demand, public expectations, and technologic advances. Regulations governing both personnel and services must be reviewed periodically to ensure that they continue to be responsive to changes in current medical practice and yet reflective of a broad consensus.

Since state regulations tend to contain minimum standards, some critics feel that such criteria are unworthy of attention because they represent only the lowest common denominator. Such critics feel that more attention should be paid to describing EMS excellence and to giving local services a goal for which to strive. Although this is certainly a valid perspective that perhaps warrants more attention, one should not underestimate the critical importance of carefully defined minimum expectations.

State minimum standards define a level of care equally applicable to urban, suburban, and even remote frontier areas. The changes in these minimum expectations over time represent the true progress of the overall EMS system. Certainly, it is fair to anticipate that areas with greater population, greater resources, or more dynamic and demanding leadership should exceed these standards. The challenge to the EMS community and to the state-level leadership is to continually upgrade the minimums as support systems and resources permit. Each time regulations are reviewed, the goal should be to forge the next most progressive consensus that will sustain continued progress without alienating or disenfranchising important participants. The decisions reached through such a process have a direct impact on the expectations for local QA efforts.

Another difficult dilemma that must be faced is the inherent conflict between both consistency and flexibility in the development and interpretation of EMS regulations. There is certainly a value to maintaining some degree of uniformity between jurisdictions. Yet, at the same time, the state should be in a position to support and encourage local initiatives. An appropriate balance must be negotiated through the regulations development process. For example, it was decided in New Mexico several years ago that EMT licensure levels should be limited to basic, intermediate, and paramedic. At the same time it was agreed that local systems could apply for "special-skills" waivers allowing them to apply for permission to locally train their providers beyond these levels. Thus, within a specific system, EMT-basics can be trained in automatic defibrillation, intermediates can intubate, and paramedics can use paralytic agents, such as succinylcholine, once an application is approved through the state EMS office.

It is the responsibility of the state EMS office to provide the leadership and direction that encourage broad participation in these critical, developmental processes. It is incumbent upon the state office to be available and responsive to feedback, as there are no "right" answers. Considered negotiation with all perspectives well represented is the best approach to ensuring that citizens will be well served.

State Roles in Quality Assurance

The state EMS office has a direct involvement in the EMS QA process. As previously discussed, it is generally mandated by law that the state adopt minimum standards, monitor performance, and take enforcement actions. This can be accomplished in various ways, ranging from the "ultimate stick" to the "productive carrot."

In the former mode the state EMS office conducts inspections and complaint investigations. As charges or concerns are substantiated, the state is empowered to take corrective or disciplinary actions. These actions generally get approved through a formal adjudicative hearing that ensures due process to those charged. In the case of an individual EMT the state may deny, suspend, or revoke licensure. In some cases the state can even initiate a civil or criminal action against the individual.

The same is true with enforcement of service standards. Penalties can range from suspending to revoking a service license to imposing a fine until corrective actions are demonstrated. Such actions are typically not the first choice for solving a QA problem, but they are absolutely necessary in some cases to protect the public.

Many state EMS offices prefer to initially play a supportive and technical assistance role in solving violation problems. If local solutions can be found that will negate or remedy a problem, everyone is better served. The state can often be much more efficient and effective by assisting local areas to operate their systems appropriately and achieve local solutions, rather than trying to solve all the problems directly from the state level. This assistance involves developing model protocols and sample guidance materials that help local systems develop plans, monitor performance, and correct their own QA problems.

This approach requires a cooperative and supportive relationship between local systems and the state EMS office. The state needs to be responsive to local requests for information and reference checks. Likewise, local services need to keep state offices apprised of problems, particularly those that aren't resolved easily. For example, a service that fires an EMT for drug or alcohol abuse may meet its needs, but the action may do nothing to help the EMT deal with his personal problem or prevent that EMT from volunteering or being hired elsewhere in the state. In addition, with mobility of personnel being fairly commonplace, contacting other state EMS offices concerning such problems can be beneficial. The state EMS office has a "need to know" in such cases so that appropriate actions can be taken to protect the entire public.

This level of communication requires trust and must be nurtured. Many state offices accomplish this by being easily accessible and meeting local needs in regard to continuing education, public information materials, legal guidance, and the like. State and local relationships can also be greatly improved by the existence of state funding to support local services and systems. In states in which the EMS community has been politically successful in obtaining dedicated EMS funding that is passed along to local areas, it fosters a stronger tie between the state and local levels.

A final and extremely important role that the state EMS office can play in the continuous quality improvement process is in recognizing excellence. The importance of identifying and rewarding outstanding performance not only reinforces excellence but also creates positive role models for other system participants. This should be happening routinely at the local level and periodically at the regional and statewide levels. Recognition should be extended not only to individual providers but also to excellent services, EMS educators, medical directors, and other system participants. It is also important to facilitate the availability of outstanding participants to provide technical assistance and support to others who are struggling. Often, a service director, instructor, or medical director is more receptive to suggestions and constructive criticism from a peer than if the same comments are made by a state official. We need to recognize and use our outstanding contributors for the good of the entire EMS system.

Summary

The state EMS office plays a legally mandated and important role in helping to ensure the delivery of quality emergency medical services. Although resources, activities, and attitudes vary considerably, state EMS offices have a critical responsibility to legally define both the scope of practice and standards of care for EMS providers and to establish minimum expectations for EMS service and system functioning. It is essential that cooperative and supportive relationships be developed and maintained to ensure that the state EMS office and local services and systems are mutually supportive in ensuring the quality of EMS.

REFERENCES

1. American Society for Testing and Materials: *Standard guide for structures and responsibilities of EMS systems organizations,* Philadelphia, 1988, The Society.
2. Metcalf W: *State and regional EMS systems.* In: *Principles of EMS systems,* Dallas, 1989, American College of Emergency Physicians.
3. National Association of State EMS Directors: The EMS office: its structure and functions, Lexington, Ky, 1988, National EMS Clearinghouse.

18

Scene Supervision of EMS

Paul E. Pepe, M.D.

Peter A. Curka, D.O.

The underlying principle of emergency medical services (EMS) is that EMS is a unique practice of medicine in which specialized physicians delegate the performance of medical acts to professional EMS personnel.[4,6,8,10] In most municipal and regional programs a single physician is designated as the physician director or "offline" medical director.[4,6] The medical community at large has come to view an EMS response as being an automatic "request for consultation" to this designated EMS physician. The nature of this consultation is to care for that medical community's patients during the brief, prehospital phase of their emergencies. In essence a public trust therefore exists that EMS personnel deliver medical care equal to the quality rendered had the delegating EMS physician been at the scene. As such, it is the obligation of a physician assuming the responsibility of medical direction for an EMS system to ensure such quality. Is this really possible, however?

At the root of medical quality always lies clinical experience coupled with the educational process. The classic principles of medical education, regardless of specialty, have always involved an apprenticeship approach. Didactics, basic skills, and clerkships may earn one a medical degree, but the apprenticeships of internship, residency, and fellowships under specialized physician mentors remain the ultimate keystones of clinical medical training.

Yet in the specialty of EMS this apprenticeship is often lacking. Instead, medical education is most often provided by EMS educators, primarily in a classroom setting. Like any other field of medicine, however, EMS also requires an apprenticeship under expert physician mentors to properly hone clinical skills and judgments in the actual patient care setting. For example, no one would send medical students out on their own to perform spinal taps on patients without on-site supervision if they had only received classroom lectures and skills testing. Unfortunately, for the most part, we still take this unguided

203

approach with emergency medical technicians (EMTs) and paramedics in many EMS systems. It must be made clear from the start that basic EMTs and paramedics also require such an apprenticeship, which should involve routine on-scene supervision and training from physicians expert in providing all levels of prehospital care.[3]

Although on-scene mentorship is an essential ingredient in proper medical education, there are other rationales for on-scene supervision. At the very least, the practical concern of having medical-legal accountability for medical acts delegated to others should be enough incentive to prompt one to directly scrutinize the prehospital care rendered. No one wants to end up in court, especially because of someone else's errors. Unfortunately, it is human nature to "cut corners." It is also human nature to develop certain bad habits, particularly when operating in a void without proper scrutiny or feedback.

In EMS, both prevention and correction of such habits usually require direct on-scene observation. That which appears to have been the provision of proper procedure, either by way of information recorded during radio communication or even by direct scrutiny on arrival at the emergency department, may not necessarily reflect potential improprieties at the scene. For example, a poor extrication procedure can be masked by subsequent meticulous spinal immobilization in the back of the ambulance. A patient may even be walked to the stretcher and then immobilized. Whether done knowingly or through ignorance, the poor scene performance not only goes unnoticed, but often such behavior is reinforced by kudos given for the way the patient presents at the hospital. The accountable medical director, however, would not have provided care in this manner had he been at the scene. Thus the original intent and purpose of this system of delegating medical care to others is lost. At one point or another, scene supervision is a must.

Ideal Structure and Function of Scene Supervision

Ideality versus Reality

Having delineated and accepted the rationale for it, the accountable physician medical director must now understand the structure and specific approach to direct on-scene supervision, as well as the realities affecting such functions in either urban or nonurban settings. In general, EMS is either a busy or a difficult practice to maintain properly.[6] In some cities a medical director may be accountable for the care of tens of thousands of patients each year within a 10- to 20-mile radius.[7] In other venues the designated medical director may only be responsible for a few hundred annual cases, but these occur in territories covering tens of thousands of square miles.[1] Despite their differences, each faces different logistic difficulties to assure proper care for each patient at each scene.

The ideal situation for an accountable physician would be to somehow directly oversee and supervise all cases, not only at the scene but also during transport and on arrival at the hospital. This ideal concept can be seen as being analogous to that of the anesthesiologist who delegates hands-on care but directly oversees each of the several nurse-anesthetists who deliver that care in each of the hospital's surgical suites. Unfortunately, in EMS the geography and case load are vastly expanded and the reality falls short of the idealistic goal. Nevertheless, adequate quality of care and supervision can still be accomplished in the majority of EMS systems if the following basic principles are met.

Structure

The logistics of EMS response and scene arrival must be predetermined and arranged in concert with the local authorities. To begin with, an EMS physician's supervisory activities are best accomplished by round-the-clock access to an emergency response vehicle, which is clearly marked (and maintained) by the local authorities.[9] Given the unpredictable nature of emergencies, this approach allows for a timely, uninhibited, and authorized response in key situations, at any time of day or night, and from any location, including home.

Other alternatives include routine "ride-alongs" accompanied by either EMS system officers and/or supervisors or directly with ambulance personnel. Unless there are no other options, responses in one's personal vehicle, with or without a "Kojak light," are discouraged. Automobile insurance coverage, personal liability, and public safety become paramount concerns of the EMS physician when using a personal vehicle.

If responding directly, the EMS physician should have specific training in emergency vehicle operation and also be familiar with the relevant policies and procedures of the jurisdictional authorities (e.g., police, fire, and state laws). Responders should possess the proper (governmental) identification required by authorities, particularly to avoid a frustrating confrontation at the very moment a patient may need them. Again, to expedite access, this concept applies to vehicular identification as well.

The EMS physician must be cognizant of street hazards that are not present in an emergency department environment, such as traffic, fire, weather, hazardous materials, weapons, and hostile crowds. The development of a "street sense" is the ability to recognize an unsafe scene and to prevent bodily harm to oneself.

The EMS physician who responds directly to the emergency scene should be equipped and prepared to deliver advanced emergency medical care. Emergencies are unpredictable, and circumstances may suddenly place the supervising EMS physician closer to the scene than the responding EMS units, especially when their arrival may be delayed as a result of geography, traffic, or even unexpected mechanical problems en route. On occasion, physicians in emergency response vehicles may happen upon or be "flagged down" at emergency scenes, even prior to activation of the EMS system.

Therefore the EMS physician should be equipped with a defibrillator and monitor (at least an automated defibrillator), oxygen delivery systems (with a bag-valve mask), and an EMS kit stocked with IV-access supplies, intubation equipment, and key drugs, such as epinephrine, lidocaine, dextrose, atropine, diazepam, nitroglycerin, and furosemide. These drugs would be the most likely to alter outcome in the interval prior to arrival of the EMS unit. In addition to classic medical supplies, thought should also be given to items such as a fire extinguisher, a high-powered flashlight, flares, binoculars, foul-weather clothing, rescue blankets, and a portable radio and cellular telephone. Depending on potential needs and the EMS system design, equipment such as splints, immobilization devices, hazardous materials references, and other drugs could also prove useful. However, the equipment catalogued above would be considered the basic minimum inventory.

Although usually not necessary, the capability of the EMS physician to perform direct patient care in the field is still clearly essential. Aside from the unexpected situations previously mentioned, a physician's ability to provide excellent prehospital care under the same conditions as any paramedic may become a key factor in establishing credibility with EMS personnel.

Dress is a matter of personal choice, but one should take into account both the patient's sensitivities and expectations, particularly when entering someone's home. For example, the appropriate respect for certain individuals may not be conveyed by wearing jeans. On the other hand, the elements and hazards likely to be encountered (e.g., blood, vomitus, and sharp objects) must also be taken into account. In addition, one's visibility on dark, rain-slickened streets should be considered.

Although a white coat with "John A. Smith, M.D." embroidered or pinned on might be an obvious choice, this approach has some disadvantages. Despite its advantages of providing visibility and conveying respect, patients have a tendency to bypass the EMTs and paramedics and start dealing with "the doctor" directly. This interferes with the evaluation process and leads to awkward deferments back to the EMS personnel. On the whole, a scrub shirt, perhaps worn with pants (and coat when needed) similar to those worn by EMS personnel, provides a more sensible approach to all the above factors. Reflective wear should be added as needed.

Function

Scene supervision, as stated previously, should be just that—supervision. Generally, it should not involve the assumption of total control of a scene. As with supervision of a medical intern, unless patient outcome truly requires direct intervention (either as a matter of assistance or to override clear mismanagement of critical medical care), scene supervision should ideally be considered an educational feedback event.

As an initial approach, the EMS physician's scene activities should center on observation while offering assistance ("What can I do for you?"). This approach not only helps one to identify the priorities and delegation talents of the EMS personnel, but it also helps to diminish their anxiety about being scrutinized. An EMS physician should be willing to do any kind of menial task needed at the scene; such humility establishes credibility, as well as a sense of empathy for the roles of others.

On occasion, scene activities may have to involve a "helpful-tip" approach, such as "Let me show you something" (or even a less patronizing gambit, such as "Let's try something here"). Speaking in the first-person plural works well.

As is the case when dealing with any type of supervisee, the egos and senses of self-esteem of EMS personnel are best dealt with through encouragement and by instilling a sense of pride in their work. An even more important incentive may be to invoke the virtues of patient care. Doing what's best for the patient is a great motivator for EMS personnel. For example, after taking a corrective action at the scene (e.g., repositioning the endotracheal tube marker from 28 cm at the front teeth up to the correct depth for the patient), you might later explain to the paramedic: "Beside the fact that *we* had to fix that right mainstem intubation for the patient's sake, I also want *you* to look 100% on target when this patient arrives at the emergency department."

In some cases, supervision might also entail scene control and direct oversight. This activity can involve double-checking for: 1) missed injuries or overlooked victims at a multicasualty scene, or 2) occult hazards, while paramedics care for the most sick and injured. Hands-on care may be inevitable in cases involving multiple victims or a severely injured individual when extra hands are necessary to expedite critical care and/or evacuation.

Nevertheless, although EMS physicians can give direct online orders at the scene that can expedite patient care, they are more effective in the role of a teacher. Future quality is more likely to be guaranteed if the paramedic or EMT is first asked, "What do you want to do now?" Although they do provide expeditious online direction, direct orders are relatively ineffective as either an evaluation or teaching tool.

Above all, EMS physicians must be role models not only in terms of the medical actions to be taken but also in terms of the behavior and the demeanor. Compassion and caring should always be paramount in the EMS physician's mind, no matter how difficult the patient or the situation. Such physician-like behavior (in the classic sense) may be the greatest teaching tool. In addition, EMS physicians must keep in mind that the example they set in providing professionalism and decorum may be needed when enthusiasm and esprit de corps occasionally become too fervent.

Ground Rules

It must be understood by all officers and administrative supervisors that medical direction and medical accountability rest with the designated medical director. Therefore no doubt should exist as to clear jurisdiction in terms of medical care.

It should be common knowledge that the medical director can (and will) show up at any given time, day or night, announced or unannounced. It should also be understood that unlike intervening physicians, EMS medical directors have unquestionable control over the medical care rendered by EMS personnel. Therefore they have the capacity and right to change any protocol or issue any medical order in any given case. However, physicians who do so without explanation (either concurrent or subsequent feedback) risk confusion or even credibility. Thus communication and education must be kept in mind (i.e., "Why did I do this?").

EMS physicians, while correcting or modifying the actions of any personnel, should also take extreme care to avoid embarrassing individuals and, perhaps more importantly, to avoid liability for all involved by announcing that a particular action or procedure was not done correctly. For example, take the case of a patient shot near the spinal area of the midback while riding on a bus who appears to be stable in condition. If the EMS personnel are observed to be preparing to walk the man off of the bus, it might be more advisable and more tactful to suggest that, "We should get a backboard for this man and make him more comfortable" (and not blurt, "Where's the backboard?!").

Liability

The EMS physician's presence at an emergency scene raises a number of medical-legal questions regarding liability and standard of care. Many states have enacted Good Samaritan laws or other legislation that may provide some protection from liability. At the same time, many of these statutes specifically exempt physicians, even when there is no expectation of remuneration. More important, if EMS is part of a physician's job responsibility, the intent of the Good Samaritan legislation may not apply. Therefore a physician would certainly present a greater target for litigation, particularly if expected to deliver prehospital care. The EMS physician's presence can also raise expectations. Unsuccessful outcomes are probably less easily forgiven than when the care providers at the scene are nonphysicians.

Still, these problems should not dissuade EMS physicians from participating in on-scene responses. Physicians can often perform an important role by directly communicating with the patient or family, and their personal presence often lends further credibility to the EMS system. Indeed, an EMS physician's presence in someone's home could be considered a house call and, if handled properly, can be extremely rewarding for the physician, the patient, the family, and the EMS system as a whole.

Above all, experienced EMS physicians eventually diminish liability for themselves (as well as for their EMS systems) by developing a unique expertise and knowledge base that is difficult to match, particularly in any courtroom.

Delegating and Developing Field Supervisory Skills

Developing Credibility

Prospective EMS physicians must gain credibility as teachers and appreciators of the differences between in-hospital and prehospital emergency care. Those who do not have clear medical authority (i.e., resident physicians on rotation or new EMS fellows) are most effective after they have become familiar to the EMS personnel, particularly in a teacher-student role. This activity, de facto, sets up a hierarchy and establishes credibility, especially if it is later balanced with firsthand knowledge of field logistics.

In addition to their didactic teaching roles, prospective EMS physicians (or even novice medical directors) need to establish credibility and rapport by active and frequent participation in prehospital care and responses. Again, such activities should be made in more of an assistance and educational capacity, at least at first. Medical authority is earned, not appointed.[8] In the streets and especially in well-entrenched EMS systems, this goal may take months (or even years) to accomplish.

Delegating Field Supervision

Although they may peak and wane, EMS activities never sleep. Therefore, when unable to provide supervision at given times, a medical director may try to delegate this responsibility directly to certain ambulance personnel. In other settings online monitoring and supervision can be delegated to assistant medical directors or, perhaps more feasibly, to shift supervisors. A small cadre of field supervisors who can effect coverage 24 hours a day on behalf of the medical director can serve as an excellent point of control.

The use of veteran paramedics as supervisory personnel who can regularly interact and learn directly from the EMS system medical director, both on-scene and didactically, is often an efficient approach to effecting full-time field supervision. Through close interaction with these few individuals, an effective, manageable span of control can be realized, particularly if operating in a large geographic jurisdiction. However, this relationship still requires the key element of apprenticeship and close physician mentorship for these select individuals, especially in the actual patient care setting. This may be achieved by routine ride-alongs with these specialized supervisory personnel.

In some EMS departments, field officers provide not only good medical care but also good leadership skills. However, the regular EMS personnel must have respect, both medically and personally, for such supervisors. Therefore mechanisms to ensure that they possess such attributes must be present in the supervisor selection process. In addition, if the responsibility of medical supervision is to be delegated, the basic principles of EMS systems (as outlined in the introduction to this discussion) must be *clearly* understood and appreciated by these direct agents of the EMS physician. In turn, such principles must be passed on to the field personnel at large.

Extent of Field Supervision

Predictable Performance

Exactly how much field supervision is enough? Field supervision is probably sufficient when the EMS physician feels reasonably confident that each individual EMS provider could be trusted to readily and safely care for the medical director's own family. At the very least, supervision should continue until each provider's individual behavior and medical performance is readily predictable.

Again, one of the principles of EMS is to delegate care to others, with the understanding that the care rendered will be the same as if the physician delegating that care was delivering it personally.[4] Therefore, to feel comfortable with the achievements of this obligation, the EMS physician should have shared a large sample of experiences with each of the individual EMS providers operating under his supervision. If necessary, EMS personnel located in distant venues might be assigned to work directly in high-volume areas for a period of time under the medical director's direct supervision.

As with anything else, EMS field supervision and evaluation can at first be intensive and continuous. Eventually, however, the relative frequency may diminish once trust (or at least predictability) is established. Nevertheless, intermittent spot checks should always be conducted to keep everyone "on their toes."

Back to the Basics

Although it may not be as appealing, one should make a conscious effort to remember that field supervisory activities should not be limited to the more "exciting" cases. In fact, a routine effort should be made to spot-check and observe the more "mundane" cases. Medical care, regardless of how basic, is still medical care.[3] Furthermore, those cases that don't involve clear-cut "life and death" actions may pose some of the most difficult decisions. Cases involving refusal or denial of service are perhaps the most compelling to supervise. Here, judgment and liability walk hand in hand. Providing a good example or delivering sound advice in such cases may, in some ways, prove to be the most important role of the EMS physician.

Summary

The entity of EMS is the practice of medicine. Ideally, the actual care provided by EMS personnel at each scene should be the same as that which would have been provided personally by the designated physician for the EMS system. To best guarantee this presumption and to best train prospective EMS personnel and physicians alike, EMS medical directors must provide on-scene education, feedback, and personal example. Because improper actions cannot be determined solely by the conditions on hospital arrival or by review of prehospital care records, scene supervision remains the true cornerstone of QA.

Therefore EMS physicians must be prepared to provide regular on-scene supervision. To do so, EMS physicians must also understand field conditions and priorities. They must be willing to establish their credibility by actively participating both in classroom training and in routine tasks in the prehospital setting. Authority is earned, not demanded. Whatever the mechanism, field response must be done in coordination with the policies and procedures of local jurisdictional authorities. Often, the use of carefully selected shift supervisors, who represent the medical director around the clock, can provide an efficient and effective instrument to realize a continuous, manageable medical chain of command.

ACKNOWLEDGMENT

The authors thank Nina Meher-Homji for manuscript preparation and the City of Houston EMS Supervisor staff, not only for the input they offered, but also for the expert guidance and tutelage they provide for scores of emergency physicians in training.

REFERENCES

1. Garnett GF, Hall JE, Johnson MS: *Rural emergency medical services.* In Kuehl AE, editor: *EMS medical directors handbook*, St. Louis, 1989, Mosby—Year Book.
2. McSwain NE: *Indirect medical control.* In Kuehl AE, editor: *EMS medical directors handbook*, St. Louis, 1989, Mosby—Year Book.
3. Pepe PE: Medical direction in basic life support, *Emergency* 22:6, 1990 (editorial).
4. Pepe PE, Bonnin MJ, Mattox KL: Regulating the scope of emergency medical services, *Prehosp Disast Med* 5:59-63, 1990.
5. Pepe PE, Copass MK: *Prehospital care.* In Moore EE, editor: *Early care of the injured*, Toronto, 1990, B.C. Decker Inc.
6. Pepe PE, Stewart RD: Role of the physician in the prehospital setting, *Ann Emerg Med* 15:1480-1483, 1986.
7. Pepe PE et al: Geographical distribution of urban trauma according to mechanism and severity of injury, *J Trauma* 30:1125-1132, 1990.
8. Stewart RD: Medical direction in emergency medical services: the role of the physician, *Emerg Med Clin North Am* 5:119-132, 1987.
9. Stewart RD, Paris PM, Heller M: Design of a resident in-field experience for an emergency medicine residency curriculum, *Ann Emerg Med* 16:175-179, 1987.
10. Subcommittee on Medical Control, Committee on Emergency Medical Services, National Research Council, Academy of Life Sciences: *Medical control in emergency medical services.* In: *Subcommittee report, conclusions and recommendations*, Washington, D.C., 1981, National Academy Press.

19

Role of the Paramedic Quality Improvement Coordinator

Jim Dernocoeur, EMT-P

As prehospital care systems have grown in complexity, the need for formalized quality assurance (QA) has also grown. The concept of overseeing, maintaining, and further refining the quality of care has always been a part of emergency medical services (EMS) systems. Yet the need to formalize this process has only recently evolved. As with any aspect of prehospital care, collaboration between prehospital care providers and medical direction is strongly needed, as only through this approach can prehospital QA become effective.

The responsibilities of the QA coordinator can be placed into two general categories. First, this person is an "environment builder" who works with the system to develop an atmosphere that fosters and promotes excellent prehospital care. The QA coordinator must ensure that prehospital personnel have the support, the medical direction, and the tools they need to do the job correctly. The system must have built-in reasons and supports (such as written "good work!" or job performance evaluations) to promote high quality care. Prehospital care providers must understand that they are able to work with (not against) the system to help direct it toward the goal of excellent care.

Second, the QA coordinator should undertake the role of "system irritant," whereby the EMS system is never allowed to become too comfortable with the current performance level. (As sand in an oyster creates a pearl, the system irritant is employed to create excellence.) The QA coordinator must evaluate every part of the system and ask, "Why do we do that? Is that effective? Is there a better way?"

Many EMS systems are plagued with the affliction of tradition, with procedures and practices based on convention rather than sound medical reasons. Once something attains the stature of being the usual and comfortable

212

thing to do, systems tend to remain static. It is the QA coordinator's role to question such practices. In fact, to promote this concept, perhaps the title *quality improvement* (QI) coordinator is more appropriate. This would lead people to question, change, refine, and move forward rather than assure the status quo.

Prehospital Care Provider's Environment and Culture

To develop the proper environment it is vital to understand the circumstances under which the prehospital care provider works. The prehospital arena is the most uncontrolled of all health-care environments. In most situations the patient's behavior must conform to the health-care provider's environment. For example, the emergency department is designed not only to provide proper patient care but also to control the patient and relatives through the triage area and the family waiting room. The patient and his family are thus somewhat constrained.

The prehospital care provider, however, must conform to the patient's environment. They must enter these surroundings to create order out of chaos that stems from a medical emergency and must be able to effectively communicate and react. Being the center of attention allows them to direct the medical care.

The prehospital care arena is sometimes hostile. Patients are often verbally and occasionally physically abusive. To make matters worse, it is not uncommon for emergency department staff to show their displeasure at the "unloading" of such unwelcome guests into their environment.

There is also a lack of follow-up in the prehospital setting. Most systems have no procedures that allow for quick and consistent follow-up on patient diagnosis and outcome. This follow-up is of critical importance to confirm appropriate care and to identify errors. In addition, prehospital care providers tend to be viewed as outsiders to the health-care system. When motivated prehospital care providers take the initiative to follow up on their patients, it is not unusual for the hospital system to resist releasing this information because of concerns about confidentiality. Thus the educational process is compromised. The only feedback is of a negative nature, as good patient care is expected. There are very few "thank you's" in most EMS systems.

Prehospital care providers themselves are an interesting group: strong willed, opinionated, independent, assertive, willing to question authority—all of which are positive attributes on the streets but are a challenge to manage. They also have a unique blend of blue-collar and white-collar thinking skills. When the prehospital care provider is working to free a patient from a crumpled automobile, clear blue-collar mechanical thinking skills are engaged. This changes, however, to white-collar skills when the provider is deciding which medication is indicated to resolve the problem discovered by the ECG patterns. Although difficult, utilization of both methods is essential.

Tools that Cultivate the Environment

Just as a plant needs the proper environment for growth, so does quality. You cannot experience quality in an environment that does not support and cultivate it. We all tend to understand this concept intellectually but fail to act on it. It is very important that the QI coordinator be active in building this environment. One of the strongest tools toward this end is mission and value statements.

From a medical perspective, mission and value statements allow a system to set its medical philosophies and values. By developing and publishing these statements, the organization establishes a foundation upon which everything

---

Mercy Ambulance Communications Center
Goals and Value Statements

Goal statement

The goal of the Mercy Ambulance Communications Center is to properly allocate system resources, to coordinate the system status management plan, and to provide prearrival instructions to allow the system to provide the best possible patient care in a professional manner.

Patient care begins not when paramedics arrive on the scene of a call, but when an emergency medical dispatcher answers the phone. Through allocation of system resources, coordination of the system status management plan, and provision of prearrival instructions, communication specialists save lives.

Value statement

For the function and growth of the communications center, Mercy Ambulance values people who:
- Place the highest priority on providing the care, support, and effort needed to help other people in time of medical need
- Provide kind care and assistance to every person with whom they come in contact
- Demonstrate that a communications specialist is a professional
- Constantly work to improve their knowledge, skills, and judgment
- Apply their craft with a positive demeanor and provide the system with leadership
- Take initiative to identify and to solve problems and work to improve and develop the field of emergency medical dispatching

For a communication specialist to perform at a competent level, he must be able to do all the above under all conditions. It takes a special person to be a communication specialist, and this procedure manual is devoted to those special people who devote their time and effort to being Mercy Ambulance communication specialists.

By permission of Mercy Ambulance, Grand Rapids, Michigan.

can be based. For these statements to help lead the organization they must be "living documents," i.e., used every day. Each time a new policy, protocol, or action is contemplated, it should be compared with the mission and value statements. If there is a discrepancy, the situation must be modified. When a prehospital care provider is in a situation that is not covered by a protocol or policy, a sound mission and value statement can serve as a guide for decision making.

Mission and value statements can also serve as guides for system development. The box on page 214 shows an example of mission and value statements. The box below is an example of a mission statement for a project. Although these assertions may at times seem lofty and unrealistic, they can be very powerful and practical. People are willing to work toward these goals if they feel that the entire system is working "in tune." Without these overt statements, it is easy for efforts to become fragmented and for providers to lose sight of the overall goal. Mission and value statements should be developed by consensus. If they are not developed, agreed upon, and accepted by everyone involved, they are of little value.

Once these statements are established, the next challenge is goal setting. These are tools that take the lofty value and mission statements and make them attainable. This allows the QI coordinator to set specific obtainable milestones to improve the medical care of the system, which can take the form of either individual or systemwide goals. The best forum for their development is a collaborative setting; prehospital care providers who become involved in this

---

Philosophy of the Clinical Improvement Program

The goal of the Clinical Improvement Program is to provide the prehospital care providers with the support, information, and equipment necessary to provide high-quality prehospital care. Through review, discussion, and exchange of ideas, clinical care and system response can be improved.

The Clinical Improvement Program is not one person telling people what to do, but is instead a process that allows for the use of collective problem solving, review, and implementation of solutions derived from a consensus of the prehospital care providers. Any part of this program will work on the following premises:

- Prehospital care personnel are skilled and intelligent people who are trying to provide patients with the best care possible
- Prehospital care personnel are worthy of trust and consistently strive to do what is appropriate for their patients
- Prehospital care providers use good judgment, including knowing their limits and using appropriate system resources when indicated
- Medical care is an art based on science. Prehospital care is provided in the most uncontrolled environment of all medical care branches.

All review processes must keep these premises in mind when trying to improve the overall performance of the system or that of a single provider.

process develop a sense of ownership regarding the goals. Once this is accomplished, the process of motivation becomes simpler.

For goals to work, they must be clearly communicated, obtainable, and stimulate the individuals and/or the system to strive for excellence. In addition, they must not only be measurable, they must, in fact, *be* measured. Each one of these components is necessary for goal setting to be successful.

Employee Screening Process

Quality prehospital care can best be provided by quality people who are well educated and supported with adequate time, resources, and authority. It is imperative that the QI coordinator be intimately involved in the selection process. Careful selection of quality personnel has the single-most lasting effect on the quality of system performance. The selection process needs to identify people who are both good employees *and* provide proper, compassionate prehospital care.

Although it is standard to check applicants for the proper credentials (such as a paramedic license), base medical knowledge is often mistakenly assumed to be sound. Therefore the QI coordinator should develop a process to check the person's ability to understand and to think. It is very important that applicants demonstrate their ability to take prehospital care concepts and apply them to solving problems in the field.

Checking an applicant's work history, driving record, references, etc., should be done by administrative personnel. The QI coordinator must be a key player in the development of the screening process that reviews basic medical knowledge, thinking and problem-solving abilities, judgment skills, and patient care philosophies. This can be achieved through a combination of a written test and interviews.

More importantly, employees must have the ability to think *and* to learn. For the most part, EMS education programs do not do a good job of preparing applicants for the field; although providers may be well trained (the "how"), they may be poorly educated (the "why"). If the applicant demonstrates the ability to learn, a strong medical orientation program can overcome a weak medical education.

Medical Orientation Program

Once the applicants have been chosen, it is important to orient them to the operational structure and medical expectations of the system. The QI coordinator needs to be involved in both of these areas.

Often, systems only provide new employees with information about how to function in the system. Seldom do they explain the medical expectations. These expectations encompass protocol knowledge, as well as philosophy and character of the prehospital care expected in a given community, and must be presented and understood by the provider in a prospective fashion. If these expectations are not presented, providers learn through periodic episodes of being "called on the carpet" for errors. This leads to negative attitudes and to the "just-do-what-will-keep-you-out-of-trouble" approach to prehospital care.

The field instructor program outlined by Pons et al[2] is an excellent example of a good medical orientation program. The Denver program educates and orients new paramedics to the system during the *screening* process to provide guidance to the expectations of the system. If new paramedics do not show adequate knowledge and skill improvement during the field instructor program, they are not allowed to continue. This process allows for field evaluation of the prospective employees, which helps identify paramedics who fare well in the interview and testing process but falter during field care.

The field instructors are experienced paramedics who have demonstrated prehospital care abilities and a desire to teach. They serve as preceptors to provide newly hired paramedics with guidance, as well as verbal and written feedback. The program is divided into three phases: orientation, education, and evaluation.

In the orientation phase the new paramedic rides as an extra crew member to observe. During this time the field instructor introduces the new paramedic to equipment, to hospitals, to protocols, and to EMS system components. In this role the new paramedic is not directly responsible for patient care.

After orientation comes the educational phase. As its name implies, the new paramedic is taught medical expectations and system function. Each spends time with the eight field instructors. After every call the field instructor verbally reviews what transpired with the new paramedic. At the end of each shift a written critique is reviewed and filed. This intensive review and feedback allows the new paramedic to learn quickly and perform in a high-volume system. The field instructors reinforce what the new person is doing correctly and also point out and improve areas of weakness.

Once the field instructors think the new paramedic is performing well (or when a maximum number of shifts have been worked), the evaluation phase begins. The field instructors work as regular partners to the new employee during this time. At the end of this phase the paramedic is released from the program in one of two ways: in "good standing," meaning that the necessary criteria have been met and the person is able to function in the system, or in "poor standing," meaning that the criteria have not been met. An individual who falls into the second category is not allowed to function in the system. In exceptional cases in which the deficiency is minor and it is believed to be correctable, the paramedic may enroll in a special program.

Feedback Tools

When most people talk about QA, they are referring to the process of standard setting, evaluation, error catching, and corrective action. When viewed from this vantage, the focus can easily become fixed on errors. This is a major cause of failure for many QA programs.

A program focused on feedback emphasizes education. The goal should be to provide the prehospital care provider with feedback on performance and educational information to improve clinical performance.

A system should have a number of feedback tools. Some of the commonly used instruments are EMS run reports, system statistics, on-scene review, radio-report reviews, and specific call-type review. Each should be used from time to time, as no single feedback tool can provide a full picture of system performance. If only one tool is used, the system improves in that area, while other parts of the system suffer. To a great extent this is what happened to paramedicine when only performance during cardiac resuscitation was examined; while cardiac resuscitation skills and statistics improved, other skills suffered.

The EMS run report review is often the first tool to be implemented when starting a QI program. Run reports provide a view of the care provided at the scene. They can be judged against system protocols and patient outcome, and system statistics can be collected.

Some of the problems encountered with EMS run report reviews stem from the fact that the data are retrospective in nature and only as good as the accuracy of the report. Additionally, they can focus more on the actual writing than the medical care rendered and can concentrate too easily on errors. When the EMS run report review is first introduced, the process is often met with anger and confusion. To minimize this the project goals and mission should be emphasized and communicated to the prehospital care providers prior to introduction of the run report review. The importance of proper documentation must be stressed, with the focus on providing performance feedback and education, not on catching errors.

Appropriate and timely response to results is crucial. Initially, the number of errors can be overwhelming and alarming, and can cause those in authority to take decisive action, typically in the form of harsh disciplinary action. This negative feedback causes the QI program to be viewed as being hostile and threatening; once this has occurred, it is *very* difficult to overcome.

It is helpful to build trust initially by seeking out cases that reflect good patient care. Feedback to the providers should point out reasons that the treatment provided was correct and appropriate. This helps people to understand that the program is not an organized witch-hunt and instead indeed supports good care. Once the program is more accepted, the more critical elements can be brought out by the review process. All critiques should be accompanied with the educational pointer necessary to promote success by the individual in the future.

It is also important to develop and publish expectations and standards prior to initiating the process. (Refer to Chapter 3 for a full discussion of standards development.) This allows individuals to understand what is expected, and it gives them a chance to improve their documentation prior to the beginning of the review process. If this is done in a collaborative atmosphere, it allows the provider to gain a sense of ownership in the program.

The box on page 219 is an example of a review standard for the CHART method (chief complaint, history, assessment, treatment, transport) of documentation. It demonstrates the desired method for documentation and serves as one standard for review. The box on page 220 is an example of a review standard for a clinical presentation. It is important to remember that no one standard

---

CHART Format Guidelines

Purpose:

To present medical information in a standard and an organized manner. This enhances readability and continuity of care.

Policy:

The narrative section of the EMS run report will be written using the CHART format. The narrative is divided into 5 sections: Cx for chief complaint, Hx for history, Ax for assessment, Rx for treatment, and Tx for transport. The information that is to be presented in each section is as follows. The information should be concise but complete.

Cx: Chief complaint — This section contains the patient's chief complaint. If trauma, state the mechanism of injury. For example, "Patient involved in auto accident, complaining of head and neck pain."

Hx: History—This section contains the history of the present illness or injury, pertinent past medical history, medications and compliance, any care provided to patient by bystanders before your arrival, and any subjective complaints made by the patient.

Ax: Assessment—In this section, document your active findings and pertinent negatives discovered during your patient examination. Most often, this will follow a methodical, head-to-toe progression. Information such as ECG and glucoscan findings should be documented in this section. The information here should consist of clear, objective findings.

Rx: Treatment—The treatment and the patient's response are documented in this section. Medications, oxygen-flow rates and method, airway care, or any other care provided are placed in this part of the report. Lung sounds after intubation are reported in this section since they are a patient response to care. If the care provided was ordered or "okayed" by the medical control physician, this should be noted here.

Tx: Transport—How the patient was moved to the stretcher, the position of patient, the mode of transport (code red or blue), and the changes in condition during transport are documented in this section.

---

covers every circumstance. Thus case reviews must be done by a person who has both the medical knowledge and field experience to fully understand the situation.

In-Field Evaluations

The in-field review process complements the EMS review process. It allows the QI coordinator to directly review field care, and it is often the best way to determine the actual care provided by the system. It is, however, very time-consuming and inefficient. There is no guarantee that the time chosen to

---

Prehospital Care Review Guidelines
Medical Problems Section

Abdominal pain

Goal of care: to identify patients with risk for hypovolemia and to provide appropriate supportive care.

Documentation and physical exam guidelines

History—Specific history needed includes: location and onset of pain; complaints of radiation to back, groin, chest or shoulder; nausea or vomiting (bloody or coffee-ground-like emesis); diarrhea, constipation, black or tar-like stools; urination difficulties or dark urine; fever; menstrual history and date of last menstrual period in females; any trauma; abnormal ingestion; medications; or recent surgical procedures.

Assessment—Specific assessment findings should include: abdominal exam findings, including tenderness, presence of guarding, distention, or pulsating mass; postural vital signs, if indicated; if patient vomits, description and estimation of volume of emesis; location of tenderness.

Treatment—Supplemental oxygen, if indicated; large-bore IVs established, fluid push as indicated, pneumatic antishock trousers, application and inflation as indicated.

Transport—Position of patient, response to therapies, any change in patient's condition en route to hospital.

---

observe will be a time with calls appropriate for clinical review. The efficiency of this QI tool is improved when numerous people in the system are used, such as field supervisors and field instructors.

Again, the focus of the program is to provide the prehospital-care provider with the feedback and education needed to improve medical care, not to find errors. This focus is consistent with the goal of a QI program. Once again, it is desirable to state performance expectations prior to program initiation.

Acting as the Liaison

A major task of the QI coordinator is to act as a liaison to the medical director, the emergency departments, the corresponding agencies, and the other parts of EMS. Through this involvement, medical care directives can be placed in the perspective of the prehospital care provider. Often, decisions are more practical as a result.

Medical direction has always been a part of the prehospital care system. Recently though, there has been a renewed interest in this role by emergency medicine physicians. The National Association of EMS Physicians, its EMS Medical Directors course, and this book demonstrate this interest. There also has been an increase in prehospital care research, which has necessitated the modification of patient care principles. It is the role of the QI coordinator to ensure that these changes are implemented with the appropriate prehospital perspective.

The QI coordinator should also bring ideas from the field to the medical director. Often, problems that hinder patient care may be apparent to the provider but obscure from the hospital's perspective. The QI coordinator must stay in contact with the field personnel to uncover such problems and use them to refine and improve the system. This allows a system to use its prehospital care providers as agents of change to improve the quality of the system.

Education

Clearly one of the most important tools of any QI program is education. Education is the best tool for promoting progress. With paramedic training programs ranging from 600 to 3000 hours and continuing education (CE) requirements varying between 0 and 100 hours a year, there is no universal agreement as to what constitutes an appropriate amount of education. Each system must determine the level of education it requires as determined by the appropriateness and level of care in the field.

Most often, the QI coordinator is directly involved in developing the CE program. It is important that this program be developed in a manner that provides prehospital care providers with the information needed to improve their level of care. It is not optimal to rehash the prehospital care provider's core curriculum time and time again; when this is the case, CE programs tend to be viewed as a bureaucratic obligation as opposed to an important tool to improve medical knowledge and care.

The CE program should strike a balance between reinforcement of basics and new knowledge. An ideal method is to formulate the program based on information from the QI data system. If there is a general need for better instruction in a particular area of care, more educational material should be reviewed in that category. Thus the information presented always has a strong level of relevance to the student, making it more interesting and easy to remember.

A good CE program can also be used to introduce new procedures, medications, or medical philosophies into the system. Resistance to change can be greatly reduced if good, solid information is presented prior to implementation.

The CE program also helps people who are experiencing performance problems. Individual problems are often based on lack of knowledge or skill. The QI coordinator can customize an individual program to address these problems.

Tools that Irritate the System

The goal of system irritation should *not* be destruction. Rather, it should be contemplation that causes the system to reevaluate what it is doing. Often, a system continues to use a procedure that no longer addresses a need.

Things must be viewed from the perspective of need, not tradition. Usually, the best way to discover a problem is simply to ask, "Why do we do that?" The answers to such questions can be very revealing. This type of question must become a part of the norm for the system. This needs to occur when a problem arises, on a scheduled basis, and during development of new programs.

Whenever a problem occurs, look at it as an opportunity for improvement. For example, if your paramedics have continual problems with figuring the proper dose of aminophylline, it is natural to question why the paramedics have this trouble. A second question to ask, however, is "Does the system need to use aminophylline at all?" Questioning the paramedic's skill is often very easy for a system to do, but to ask itself if the system is doing the right thing can be far more difficult. The QI coordinator should maintain a perspective and always reflect on how the system can be modified to eliminate such problems.

Most policies should receive this type of questioning on a scheduled basis. Medical protocols are a good example. Since the field of prehospital care is always changing, it is important for protocols to be reviewed regularly for updating. This allows systems to rid themselves of unneeded procedures and policies.

Becoming a Quality Improvement Coordinator

The proper career path to become a QI coordinator has yet to be established. At present, there are a number of definitions and job descriptions for this position. It is unclear exactly what type of background and experience is necessary and desirable. From personal experience I would suggest that the QI coordinator demonstrate the following abilities:

Interpersonal communication skills—The bulk of the work a QI coordinator does is based on communicating concepts, praise, and concerns. To be successful, that person must have the ability to listen and to integrate the ideas of other people.

Analytical skills—This person must have the ability to review data and to develop an understanding of system performance. This individual also needs to be able to develop a system that collects the data necessary to capture an understanding of system performance.

Teaching skills—Often, the best way to react to a problem is to teach the person a better perspective. Because of this, teaching skills in both a one-on-one situation and as a group are necessary. This person should have experience in these roles before taking on the job of QI coordinator.

Management skills—This person often has a number of projects that must be managed. Organizational and delegation skills are very useful. This person needs to be able to work with and to encourage others to work toward improving quality.

Clinical skills—Much of the work of a QI coordinator is to ensure adequate clinical performance of the system. Without an intimate knowledge of clinical skills, this is difficult to do. This person should have a good foundation of medical knowledge and prehospital care experience. A strong working knowledge of the environment and the subtleties of the field is essential. One cannot expect a person to ride a few shifts and gain the level of understanding of the field necessary to function as a system's QI coordinator. Field experience also lends a great deal of credibility among the field personnel.

Summary

Both the EMS systems and the needs of their QA programs have grown in complexity. Because of this, the role and the tools of the paramedic QI coordinator need to be clearly defined and understood. The role of the paramedic QI coordinator should be viewed as being an environment builder and system irritant. To understand the tools needed to develop a quality environment, there needs to be a good understanding of the working environment of prehospital care providers. Once that is done, other tools— mission statements, value statements, goal-setting, employee screening, orientation programs, feedback, statistics, and education—can be well used.

Being the system irritant means causing the system to reevaluate continually and to improve every process. EMS systems tend to become very complacent and to develop habits that no longer help to improve overall performance. The paramedic QI coordinator needs to look at each process in a system and ask, "Why do we do that?" With this type of questioning, problem areas can be identified and improved.

The role and function of the QI coordinator are very complex and important to the growth of any EMS system. Most importantly, the QI coordinator must be genuinely viewed as being an integral part of the system. It's not *just* a department that takes care of quality. The focus on quality must be interwoven into everything that is done within the organization. Each new project or idea needs to be checked against the system's mission and value statements. The QI coordinator helps to see that the system stays on track.

REFERENCES

1. Davidow WH, Uttal B: *Total customer service: the ultimate weapon,* New York, 1989, Harper & Row.
2. Pons PT et al: The field instructor program: quality control of prehospital care, the first step, *J Emerg Med* 2:421-427, 1985.

20

Prehospital Research and Quality Assurance

Donald M. Yealy, M.D.

On the surface, prehospital research and quality assurance (QA) appear to conflict: a clinical research trial varies treatment among patients to detect a difference, whereas QA attempts to ensure there is no difference in care among patients. However, research and QA share many characteristics and can be performed simultaneously. This chapter highlights the basic features of good emergency medical services (EMS) research and lists the common ground, conflicts, potential benefits, and pitfalls of prehospital research as QA.

Basic Research Design

Although cellular and animal experiments are common in biomedical research, EMS research largely focuses on the investigation of humans, including both patients and prehospital care providers. If an intervention is introduced for study, it can range from drug or device use (e.g., thrombolytics or cervical immobilization equipment) to determining a more efficient method of managing resources (e.g., different levels of response). Research trials can be performed using a variety of formats. Each design has its strengths and flaws; the researcher must choose between the virtues of less-sophisticated but more "do-able" designs versus more detailed and difficult designs, with no one choice being correct. The reader is referred to other works for a more "nuts-and-bolts" approach to research design and implementation.[2,3,5,9,10]

All research, including EMS research, can be broadly divided into two categories: observational and experimental studies. In observational studies, events are monitored and analyzed without making any attempt to manipulate or alter the outcome. Traditional QA often follows this format; an area of concern is identified, monitored, and analyzed without initially trying to influence the event. For example, the administration of a specific drug by paramedics can be monitored and analyzed to uncover the patterns that govern its use. Although this design is simple, it has limited ability to answer any questions, and is best used to identify areas in need of further study. Thus observational designs serve as a good first step in the investigation of a topic.

Experimental designs introduce an intervention and then monitor its effect on the outcome. In fact, most experimental designs in all human research are "quasi-experiments," a term coined to reflect the lack of absolute control over all variables that is needed to create a true experiment.[2,3] Although animal and human trials seek to control all interventions and treatments, in practice this cannot be accomplished. Often, we fail to recognize events or factors that may influence outcome and thus fail to control these events. True experiments occur only when all variables influencing outcome are identified and under strict control, and when random enrollment of subjects into treatment groups is performed. For the sake of simplicity, however, the terms *experiment* and *experimental design* are used to denote any attempt to measure outcome after an intervention, recognizing the implicit flaw in human trials that "comes with the territory."

In general, observational studies are easier to perform than experimental studies, but the latter allow the investigator to better determine any cause-and-effect relationship. Prehospital research, especially disaster research, lends itself to observational studies since many events are sporadic, beyond control, and unpredictable. However, events that occur more frequently or those subject to some control are better studied using an experimental design once a problem is identified.

Common and Divergent Characteristics of Prehospital Research and Quality Assurance

Data Analysis

In addition to design traits, prehospital QA and research share methods and language. Data from QA and research trials are initially evaluated and reported using descriptive statistics; these help paint a compact and organized picture of what happened during the observational or experimental period. Often, some measurement of the central tendency (or the "average") is reported, such as the mean, median, or mode, as is a measurement of the variability of the individual scores (the standard deviation and range).[9,11] When reporting on categoric or exclusive events (such as patients who survived or died; are male or female; improved, worsened, or experienced no change), frequency tables and cumulative totals help to organize the results. Certain data are easier to interpret if grouped into more meaningful sets, such as percentiles or confidence intervals.[5,14]

Analytic statistics are used in both QA and research to compare groups to better determine if any difference truly exists.[1,5,9,13] The major goal of analytic evaluation is to provide a mathematic estimate of the likelihood that any observed difference could have been the result of chance alone (and thus not a true treatment effect). This mathematic probability estimate is communicated as the familiar p value. The p value answers the question for an investigator, "How likely is it that my data are fooling me and chance alone could account for any differences?" When a chance event is erroneously thought to be a result of a treatment effect, a Type I (or alpha) error is committed. One can never eliminate the possibility of a Type I error, but before collecting and analyzing data, the level accepted should be set. Generally, if the risk of misinterpreting chance effects as a treatment result is 1 in 20 (0.05) or less, the results are considered scientifically acceptable; p values (which are probability estimates of this error based on obtained data) less than or equal to this are considered to be "significant."

If no difference is noted between two or more groups, analytic statistics can help define the Type II (or beta) error. A Type II error occurs when a true treatment effect was missed because of inadequate sampling. Analogous to the p value is the power calculation. This estimates the likelihood that a difference could have been detected given the study population and variability. Thus it answers the question, "How hard did we look for a difference?" The power estimation is related to the Type II error and is equal to $1 -$ beta error. By convention, the acceptable Type II error is 1 in 5 (or 0.20, with power = 0.80) or less (i.e., lower Type II error rate or higher power estimate).

Contrary to popular belief, analytic testing does *not* evaluate the clinical importance of the observations, nor does it define any cause-and-effect relationships.[1,13] Low p values and high power estimates do not signify more important observations, but merely the probability of that occurrence (i.e., an estimate of the likelihood of an erroneous conclusion). There are a multitude of analytic tests available to compare data, and the choice is usually driven by the type of data collected and the specific comparison sought. The reader is referred to a more detailed source for further details.[2,3,5,9-11]

Clinical Features

Aside from language and data analysis, EMS research and QA have another common goal: improving patient care. Other secondary goals shared are increased understanding of the dynamics of prehospital care, uncovering harmful or ineffective practices, and better tailoring of treatments to needs.[6,7] Often, there is no distinction between prehospital research and QA.[8] For example, studying the best method of assuring quality care (computer-assisted chart audit versus manual,[16,17] online versus offline medical command) constitutes both research and QA. Similarly, investigating the frequency of complete assessment and documentation of vital signs in a specific patient population (e.g., trauma patients[15]) may provide information useful to QA and research programs.

Prehospital research and QA goals appear to diverge as the sophistication of the design increases. Observational, cross-sectional, and retrospective designs (especially chart reviews) are often used to track the quality of care and to investigate a particular topic. These designs all suffer from a limited ability to draw strong cause-and-effect relationships but still can assess the quality of care. Because of these limitations, observational and cross-sectional designs are best used to generate and define, rather than answer questions or solve problems. A retrospective study can then be performed to further define the question and to provide some data regarding the answer. When an event or outcome is rare (e.g., survival from asystole), a retrospective design may be the most practical method of evaluating a problem.

A prospective, randomized, controlled (PRC) design can provide data capable of defining cause-and-effect, particularly when coupled with blinding and a placebo control. However, PRC trials require actions that appear contradictory to the goals of QA. For example, the field provider must administer a specific treatment to a patient based in part on a factor outside of the provider's control (the randomization table or a coin-flip.) In a "blinded" study, the provider does not know what treatment is being given to patients. Also, certain specific measurements must be taken at set time intervals, even if inconvenient. Most troublesome to QA and field personnel is the possibility that one group of patients will receive an inferior or less optimal treatment (although a harmful treatment should never be investigated). This raises ethical and liability issues. These conflicts can be mitigated if close attention is paid to proper design and implementation.

Prospective Trials and Quality Assurance

Before conducting a prospective field trial, the available data and medical literature should suggest that each treatment (including a placebo) has an equal chance of benefiting each subject. Although final analysis may suggest one treatment is superior to another, any knowledge of this before the trial obviates the need for an investigation. Usually, investigators believe that one treatment is more or less beneficial; this belief, however, does not constitute scientific knowledge of that effect. Placebos, although intended to be pharmacologically inactive[4,12], are often associated with a subjective or objective benefit; it is this fact that justifies their use in trials, especially in nonlife-threatening diseases. When a scientifically proven standard of care exists, it should be used as the control agent in a PRC trial, and the use of a placebo is not justified.

Although the PRC design does not allow the provider to choose which treatment each patient is given, quality care can be provided if the selection criteria for enrollment are clear, the ability to terminate experimental treatment is available, and the method of unblinding treatment is used. These steps help ensure that only those patients with a similar disease are studied and no subject enrolled is likely to experience harm. Having a simple and clear mechanism to unblind treatment ensures that the clinical care of each patient can be tailored to need if a problem arises. Finally, the data accumulated should be analyzed at defined intervals by a person(s) not directly involved with patient enrollment. This identifies any inappropriate enrollment of subjects or unexpected harm. These preliminary data may require the trial to be modified or (if compelling) terminated without exposing more subjects to a suboptimal or harmful treatment.

Benefits and Pitfalls in Prehospital Research: A Quality Assurance View

Although well-designed prehospital research can provide the field and administrative personnel with many benefits, certain pitfalls must be avoided. Identifying these traps before and after undertaking a study can help create research that assists in the task of QA and may allow data initially collected for QA purposes to be presented to colleagues as formal research. A detailed discussion of protocol development, funding, informed consent, and internal review board approval is beyond the scope of this text; the reader is referred to other sources for this information.[*]

Study Design

The conclusions reached from research or QA data depend highly on the reasons for which the data were obtained; information obtained from an unfocused investigation produces data that are unfocused and difficult to interpret. The investigator must choose a specific question to answer or a specific problem to solve; in research jargon, a *hypothesis* is generated. This specific question (s) is essential to both research and QA investigations. The hypothesis statement is a declarative thought to be proven or disproven; in the case of the latter, the null hypothesis states that no difference exists between two or more treatments.

Although useful information on one topic can be gleaned from a trial intended to answer a question on an unrelated topic, this is the exception rather than the rule. Good research and good QA are focused: ask a specific question first, and then design a trial that can answer that question. One helpful exercise is to write, in one or two succinct sentences, what your question(s) is before starting any research or QA endeavor. This may be modified later, but starting with a clear, focused question improves the quality of the design and the data collected.

After creating a specific research question, the current literature must be reviewed, with at least two computerized searches followed by a manual review of the cited references. Often, the question is answered in a previously published work (obviating the need for a trial), or information concerning unanticipated problems may become apparent (allowing the design to be adjusted to avoid these.) For both QA and research investigations this search eliminates the need to "reinvent the wheel" when a particular area is to be studied. When the search

[*]References 2, 3, 5, 9, 10, 18, 19.

is complete, the investigator should be an expert on the topic and capable of writing a review article.

Prior to developing a protocol, especially if a PRC trial is contemplated, the help of a statistician should be sought if the investigator is not experienced in this area. Aside from formulating a strategy for data tabulation and analysis, the statistician can help determine the size of the study population needed. Sometimes it becomes obvious that the question asked requires such a large number of subjects that it cannot be done in a timely or economic fashion. This consult may prevent the investigator from performing a study that, however well designed, cannot provide the information desired or, worse, provides misleading information. It also helps prevent unnecessarily enrolling too many subjects.

Before asking the consultant how many patients should be enrolled, the investigator should decide which measurements are most important and how much difference between groups is clinically important. These two factors should guide the sample-size determination; often, investigators decide these after seeing the results of mathematic manipulations. When these clinical features are identified after the fact, the results of the trial may reach statistical significance without having any clinical significance.

Practical Considerations

During the writing and implementation of a protocol, it is wise to involve those who will be responsible for data collection and subject treatment. Often, a street-smart emergency medical technician (EMT) or paramedic can provide practical tips to help streamline the protocol. The inclusion of these providers in the design and implementation of a trial can also help build support from within the system. Finally, these colleagues can aid the principal investigator in "keeping the ball rolling" after data collection begins, especially if any difficulties arise. Studies without this type of involvement may encounter difficulties because of perceived or real shortcomings in the protocol identified by the field providers.

In a similar fashion the investigators must continually seek input from the field providers and answer any concerns raised as the trial proceeds. Frequently scheduled meetings that include the supervisors and field providers are quite helpful in identifying concerns or problems before they mushroom. In the absence of this ongoing contact, enrollment and data collection are perceived as being tasks without benefit.

Whenever economically feasible and practical, the person collecting the data should not be responsible for providing the clinical care. Having a research assistant with sufficient medical knowledge ride-along to ensure that subjects are enrolled and protocol is followed improves the quality of the data collected. This approach, although costly and often impractical, reduces the perception of "extra work" on the part of the field providers. Often, students, off-duty medics, or others can perform this task through a voluntary or stipend arrangement.

Regardless of who collects the data, the form used should be simple and nonredundant with the prehospital care record. Organizing the sheet so that data are collected and recorded at the time of each intervention and measurement, and using a checklist or electronic bar-coding system whenever possible, helps improve the quality and consistency of the information. A cumbersome form that requires redundant information or lengthy prose produces inconsistent data that are often incomplete and hard to interpret. It cannot be overstated that although EMS personnel appreciate participating in most studies, no one appreciates extra paperwork.

Benefits of Research

The first benefit of prehospital research is that data can be obtained to help improve the care of those treated in the future. Another benefit is the quality of care provided to subjects in the present. Contrary to the perception that care varies in a PRC study and some patients experience a worse outcome, in fact, care tends to be improved for all patients.

Subjects treated within a well-designed protocol generally receive high-level, homogeneous care. This is because the knowledgeable investigator tries to control all outside influences and optimize ancillary treatments and actions to better detect the actual effect of the study intervention. Data from inpatient research suggest that many patients within a experimental trial demonstrate subjective and objective improvement to a greater degree than those with similar diseases treated outside of a study protocol.[10] Such benefits can occur even when subjects are randomized to an intervention that eventually is determined to be less effective than another; this is the result of a well-defined, consistent treatment plan (including ancillary treatments not being manipulated for study purposes) coupled with vigilant monitoring of benefit or harm. To reap these advantages the investigator must carefully plan the trial such that the study intervention and ancillary care are practical, medically sound, clearly defined, and monitored. A poorly designed and implemented prospective trial does not produce this benefit and may become a QA liability.

When a prospective prehospital trial is well designed, closely monitored, and successful in answering a question, others beside current and future patients benefit. All involved gain insight into the pathophysiology of the problem studied. Additionally, the research authors and the system gain academic recognition. The field providers derive satisfaction from seeing "science in the field" impact care. The people within the system also learn that medical practice is dynamic and gain a better understanding about the natural evolution and change required to continually improve care. Thus clinical skills, judgment, and esprit de corps are positively influenced.

Pitfalls in Interpreting Data

Observational, cross-sectional, and retrospective designs can uncover shortcomings in patient care and resource allocation and may help identify areas for prospective research. These designs do not interfere with clinical care as it is delivered, so the diligence of the investigator is usually the only stumbling block to completing the trial. Thus these designs rarely conflict with QA and serve as useful tools in documenting the type of care provided. Aside from the cause-and-effect shortcomings outlined previously, these designs are prone to challenges based on the validity of the data recorded and the conclusions reached. Data from prospective designs may also fall prey to concerns about validity.

Internal validity refers to the truth within a study. Simply put, internal validity says the investigators measured what they thought they were measuring. For example, if a change in Glasgow coma score (GCS) is used to assess the effect of a trauma-care treatment, scores should be taken over time by the same observer or observers with similar training. Comparing GCS at the scene (estimated from an EMT-written prehospital care record or calculated by the scene EMT) with those judged by an attending physician in the emergency department may be invalid; any change can be the result of a treatment effect, different observers, charting anomalies, or a combination of these factors. Problems with internal validity are best sought and addressed prior to data collection.

External validity refers to the ability to generalize results and conclusions from a study population with other systems or geographic areas. Some data are system specific, whereas others are reflective of features shared by many systems. QA projects that are crafted into research trials after the fact are prone to problems with limited external validity. For example, poor outcome from out-of-hospital cardiac arrest may reflect problems within that system alone (such as a faulty defibrillator, long response times, a unique patient population). Although this information is useful within the system as a QA tool, it has a limited external validity. There are no rules to determine the external validity of collected data and conclusions; the investigator should ask before and after the trial, "What do my observations mean to others?"

Finally, data from *all* patients enrolled in a trial must be analyzed, not just from those who completed the protocol. This analysis, based on "an intention to treat," helps uncover benefits or harm that might have been missed if only those who completed the protocol were examined. For example, a prehospital PRC trial investigating the effect of inhaled nitrous oxide and/or oxygen for traumatic pain that only analyzes those who could complete a minimum 5-minute course of treatment may overlook side effects or other harms experienced by those who refused further participation after 1 to 2 minutes.

Summary

Prehospital research and QA can exist and flourish together if each investigation is carefully planned and common pitfalls are avoided. Well-designed EMS research shares many goals and features with QA, and should not interfere with good patient care in the field. The final results of good EMS research and QA are improvement of care and more efficient allocation of resources.

ACKNOWLEDGMENT

The author thanks Thomas J. Greene, M.D., and James J. Menegazzi, Ph.D., for their assistance and support.

REFERENCES

1. Browner WS, Newman TB: Are all significant p values created equal? *JAMA* 257:2459-2463, 1987.
2. Campbell DT, Stanley JC: *Experimental and quasi-experimental designs for research,* Boston, 1963, Houghton Mifflin Co.
3. Cook TD, Campbell DT: *Quasi-experimentation: design and analysis issues for field settings,* Boston, 1979, Houghton Mifflin Co.
4. The Coronary Drug Project Research Group: Influence of adherence to treatment and response of cholesterol on mortality in the coronary drug project, *N Engl J Med* 303:1038-1041, 1980.
5. Elston RC, Johnson WD: *Essentials of biostatistics,* Philadelphia, 1987, F.A. Davis Co.
6. Gibson G: Emergency medical services: the research gaps, *Health Serv Res* 9:6-21, 1974.
7. Gibson G: EMS evaluation: criteria for standards and research designs, *Health Serv Res* 11:105-111, 1976.
8. Holyrod B, Knopp R, Kallsen G: Medical control, quality assurance in prehospital care, *JAMA* 256:1027-1031, 1985.
9. Hulley SB, Cummings SR, editors: *Designing clinical research,* Baltimore, 1988, Williams and Wilkins.
10. Iber FL, Riley WA, Murray PJ: *Conducting clinical trials,* New York, 1987, Plenum Medical Book Co.
11. Menegazzi JJ, Yealy DM: Methods of data analysis in the emergency medicine literature, *Am J Emerg Med* 9:225-227, 1991.
12. Pasternak SJ, Paris PM: *Placebo therapy.* In Paris PM, Stewart RD, editors: *Pain management in emergency medicine,* Norwalk, Conn, 1988, Appleton & Lange.
13. Riegelman R: The importance of significance and the significance of importance, *Postgrad Med* 66:119-124, 1979.
14. Simon R: Confidence intervals for reporting results of clinical trials, *Ann Intern Med* 105:429-435, 1986.
15. Spaite DW, et al: A prospective evaluation of prehospital patient assessment by direct in-field observation: failure of ALS personnel to measure vital signs, *Prehosp Disast Med* 5:325-334, 1990.
16. Swor RA, Bocka JJ, Maio RF: A paramedic peer-review quality assurance audit, *Prehosp Disast Med* 6:321-326, 1991.
17. Swor RA, Hoelzer MH: A computer-assisted quality assurance audit in a multi-provider EMS system, *Ann Emerg Med* 19:286-290, 1990.
18. Yealy DM, Scruggs KS: Study design and pre-trial peer review in EMS research, *Prehosp Disast Med* 5:113-118, 1990.
19. Yealy DM, Scruggs KS, Weiss LD: Informed consent in prehospital research, *Am J Emerg Med* 5:560, 1989.

21

Using Cardiac Arrest Data to Evaluate the EMS System

Ronald F. Maio, D.O.

A primary goal in the development of prehospital care systems was the successful treatment of out-of-hospital cardiac arrests resulting from cardiovascular disease.[4,15] In a monumental study, Eisenberg et al [2] demonstrated the effectiveness of paramedic care in treating out-of-hospital cardiac arrest patients and provided extensive information regarding structural and process measures that are related to successful outcome. Many of those process measures have since been adopted as performance criteria for EMS systems, regardless of the nature of the medical problem. Recently, it has been demonstrated that paramedic treatment of out-of-hospital cardiac arrest is more cost-effective than organ transplantation or curative chemotherapy for acute leukemia.[20]

Although treating cardiac arrests accounts for only a small percentage of advanced life support (ALS) ambulance runs, it remains the only clinical entity for which prehospital care has been scientifically demonstrated to save lives. This chapter discusses how an event that represents only a small portion of a system's activity can be used as an important measure of its quality of care.

Rationale for Using Cardiac Arrests in Quality Assurance

Evaluation of an entire EMS system is a costly and time-consuming process. Evaluation efforts may be efficiently used by focusing on one or several specific "tracer" medical conditions to assess the care rendered. These tracers should have the following characteristics: 1) be an important event, 2) have a clear case definition, 3) have a measurable outcome, 4) have a straightforward intervention, 5) have an intervention that has an effect, 6) be sufficiently prevalent to permit the collection of adequate data.[3,12] The treatment of out-of-hospital cardiac arrests by paramedics is currently the only prehospital intervention for which information exists that clearly links structure, process, and outcome. This prehospital intervention fulfills all the criteria for a tracer condition.

Eisenberg[7] has stated that system evaluation of prehospital cardiac arrest (PHCA) is "the best outcome evaluation of an EMS system's performance." Cardiac arrest stresses all the system's components, from access to arrival at receiving hospitals: it is the time-critical event within that system.[17] It crosses traditional component boundaries to assess how individual components are integrated to provide care. Recommended performance standards for EMS systems are based on PHCA survival.[18,19] However, evaluation of PHCA must be done locally; the extreme variability in current reporting methods and configuration of EMS systems in North America precludes EMS systems from assuming that performance criteria with favorable outcomes in another system automatically result in locally favorable outcomes.[10]

Not only can evaluating cardiac arrests tell us something about the overall quality of our system, it can also be used to monitor performance of critical skills by providers, such as intubation and IV insertion. Additionally, we can use our evaluation data to help us investigate new or alternative management strategies. For instance, if the current survival rate for cardiac arrests is known, the benefits of proposed new therapies and protocols can be objectively evaluated.

Methods

Important variables need to be defined in evaluating the treatment of cardiac arrest. The Ustein II Conference developed a template particularly well suited for research comparing different systems.[5] Parameters were identified for system evaluation, as well as for research. Currently, however, it may be impossible for many systems to be able to obtain all the data points recommended by Ustein, either prospectively or retrospectively. In general, it should be possible to obtain information regarding the following critical variables:

1. Patient age
2. Presenting rhythm
3. If the arrest was witnessed
4. If bystander CPR was performed
5. If patient was admitted to hospital
6. Discharge status (patient discharged alive?)
7. Critical time intervals (e.g., system activation to ambulance arrival and definitive care rendered)
8. If the arrest was a result of cardiovascular disease

Polnitsky and Eisenberg[5,9,11,16] have both proposed standard definitions for these variables. The Ustein recommendations are considered by some to be the "gold standard" for variable definition. Yet whatever definition is used, it must be recorded and stored in a written and easily retrievable format, as in the first box on page 235.

Another task to be accomplished prior to data gathering is to develop decision rules to guide abstractors in interpreting information on ambulance run sheets

Example of Standard Definitions of Data Abstraction

1. *Cardiac arrest from cardiovascular disease:* An unresponsive, apneic, pulseless state confirmed by a paramedic or EMT and primarily caused from a cardiac etiology.
2. *Witnessed arrest:* One that is either observed or the collapse directly heard, such that a bystander is immediately aware that a rapid and unexpected loss of consciousness took place.
3. *Unwitnessed arrest:* One in which a collapsed patient is discovered, with an indeterminate time interval since collapse.
4. *Bystander:* Someone not actively on duty with a police, fire, or ambulance agency.
5. *CPR:* Attempts at artificial respiration *and* chest compressions.
6. *Ventricular fibrillation:* Totally disorganized depolarization and contraction of small areas of ventricular myocardium with no effective ventricular pumping activity. The monitor pattern shows a fine to coarse zigzag pattern without discernible P waves or QRS complexes.

Example of Decision Rules for "Rhythm" Provided to Abstractors

1. If the rate is less than 60, the rhythm is bradycardia.
2. If the initial rhythm is noted to be "fine ventricular fibrillation" or "fine ventricular fibrillation asystole," the rhythm is asystole.
3. If an "agonal rhythm" is noted, the rhythm is asystole.
4. If an "idioventricular rhythm" is noted and it is not described as being "slow," the rhythm is EMD.
5. If a patient being rhythm-monitored has an arrest, the rhythm used is the first one noted at the time of pulselessness and apnea.
6. If an arrest patient has a pacemaker and only pacer spikes are noted with no electrical capture, the rhythm is asystole. If a pulseless patient has a pacemaker present with electrical capture, the rhythm is EMD.

(see second box on this page). It cannot be assumed that consistency among different abstractors can be accomplished using only written variable definitions.[14] Decision-rule development is often a dynamic process with most rules being written prior to and the remaining during data collection. Using both definitions and decision rules aids in ensuring consistency in data collection. During the analysis phase this careful documentation of definitions and data abstraction ensures that differences in outcome between different years or different systems are not a result of methodological variations.

A critical variable not normally collected by EMS systems is the interval from scene arrival until definitive care is delivered. In at least one study[1] this interval has been shown to equal the response interval of the ambulance and may have dramatic effects on patient survival. Other variables that may be added are the type of procedures done and whether they were successfully completed. Thus performance of critical skills in a system (e.g., IV insertion and intubation) can be measured from cardiac arrest data.

Information should be collected that identifies the geographic area where the arrest took place. This allows for analysis of geographic variation within the system for either performance or outcome. It also can provide information regarding the efficient use of resources. Demographic information relating to race or income level can also provide important information regarding variation in performance or outcome measures.

Most systems abstract information from ambulance run sheets and contact emergency departments and medical records departments to get outcome information. These data are then numerically coded and entered into the computer. A microcomputer with a 20- to 40-megabyte hard drive is sufficient for most systems. Current commercially available data base or spreadsheet programs can be used for data collection and initial analysis. The files from these programs can be imported into microcomputer statistical software packages if more sophisticated analysis is desired.

Interpreting Results

The goal of QA is to take information regarding the structure, performance, and outcome of a system and provide feedback to practitioners and planners so that this information can be used to improve the system. The information gathered for QA of cardiac arrest cases can be used in numerous ways. Cummins[11] recommends that discharge alive from witnessed ventricular fibrillation (V-fib) be reported as the main outcome measure. This represents the subgroup of PHCAs most likely to benefit from treatment. Using witnessed V-fib patients as the denominator minimizes the problem of variability of protocols and case definition between systems or annually within a system. If one uses the basic data elements previously described, one is not limited to just reporting or analyzing witnessed V-fib. For example, it would be possible to determine survival rate for all cardiac arrests or analyze an intermediate outcome measure, such as admission to hospital.

Data regarding procedural performance can be presented in a summary format. Explicit criteria can be developed to flag certain cases for implicit review. For example, cardiac arrest patients who were not successfully intubated, had prolonged times to definitive care, or were treated with automatic defibrillators could be implicitly reviewed for overall care rendered. Individual provider experience and performance, as well as systemwide performance, could also be evaluated.

Determining how these data will be used to improve care can be extremely complex and requires a balanced evaluation of outcome and process measures. Setting a goal or outcome criteria to be met can be an important step in the analytical process. Some investigators recommend that a discharge-alive-from-hospital rate of 20% for all patients having a witnessed V-fib arrest is an attainable goal for most EMS systems in the United States. Whether or not a system meets this outcome criterion lets it know how it's doing, but does not provide any insight into why it did not meet the criterion or if it is possible to improve even if its outcome criterion is met.

To gain such insights, process measures must also be evaluated. The most common performance criterion used by EMS systems is a response interval of 8 minutes or less for 90% of all cardiac arrest patients. Cummins et al[5] have pointed out the importance of clearly defining the time interval one is evaluating and define an *ALS response time interval* as being the interval between receiving the call for aid and when the ambulance arrives at the scene.

If, for example, a system has a 10% survival rate for witnessed V-fib and 60% of the cardiac arrest patients have a response time interval of 8 minutes or less, a specific process measure has been identified as a possible reason for not meeting outcome criteria. The system can then develop strategies to overcome the specific performance deficiency (or several deficiencies) and anticipate what the results on outcome will be. If, on the other hand, response time interval data are excellent yet survival rates are still less than expected, further evaluation might focus on other components of the system (e.g., dispatch, access through 9-1-1, bystander CPR, or time to arrival of first responder) as areas for concern.

The complexity of the data analysis increases rapidly when one considers multiple process measures, which underscores the need for outcome-based evaluations. For example, what if along with a poor response time interval, the witnessed bystander CPR rate for a system is 5%? Other systems have documented much higher bystander CPR rates and have identified this variable as being an important predictor of survival. The system has to prioritize where to make changes and at what cost. Regardless of the steps a system takes, it can always use outcome as an indicator of the effects of those changes.

Analyzing geographic and demographic variations of the frequency, characteristics, and outcome of cardiac arrest cases can also prove valuable. For example, these variations may be used to determine where automatic defibrillators should be used for optimal effect. Poorer outcomes among different socioeconomic or racial groups may reflect inadequate education of these populations regarding system access, difficulties associated with the structures in which they live (e.g., high-rise apartments with poorly functioning elevators), or real or perceived dangers posed to providers when quickly accessing the patient.

A compelling use of outcome data is that it may be used to justify and quantify the effect of expenditures to improve outcome. An analysis of the effect of increased use of automatic defibrillators in Michigan's Washtenaw County based on response time interval data for each fire district estimated that adding five automatic defibrillators in one urban fire district would result in 10 to 20 more lives being saved over a 5-year period at a cost of approximately $1912 to $3823 per life saved. This information was shared with the municipal authority, which used it to justify new budget requests.[13]

Comparing the outcome of one system to another must be done with extreme caution. Differences in survival could be due to differences in the geographic characteristics of the systems or differences in variable definition and data collection. For example, the Washtenaw/Livingston (W/L) Counties' EMS system in southeastern Michigan encompasses the urban areas of Ann Arbor and Ypsilanti but also includes large, sparsely populated rural areas. It would be inappropriate to compare the overall outcome of that system with data from Milwaukee or Tucson. On the other hand, it would be appropriate to compare outcome in the urban areas of the W/L EMS system with those of other urban areas throughout the nation. Other factors, such as criteria for case entry (e.g., are cardiac arrests that occur after respiratory failure of unknown etiology included?) may also vary, resulting in very different survival rates.

Limitations

One of the major stumbling blocks in procuring outcome data is obtaining cooperation from hospitals. Systems must secure agreement with participating hospitals to submit data. Having representatives from all the system's hospitals on the QA committee or a data management committee should minimize the problem. Hospitals and providers also need to trust that data will not be publicly distributed in an inappropriate forum, reflecting poorly on a specific hospital or agency.

Another concern involves the frequency of cardiac arrests in a given system, which average two to three PHCAs per day per million population.[9] Will evaluation in a system that typically responds to 25 cardiac arrests per year be any less valuable or efficient than a system that responds to 250 arrests per year? A low frequency of cardiac arrests in a system does not detract from the fact that treatment of that condition is a major reason for that system existing. Also, in performing QA one is not as concerned with sample size as if implementing a clinical trial. Information that may not result in statistical significance can still be of great value in assessing the clinical process and the outcome. There is no reported minimum frequency of cardiac arrests that would render evaluation of their treatment no longer productive.

Another issue is efficiency: usually, systems with a smaller cardiac arrest volume are less likely to have funding or personnel available to perform data collection. The fact that these resources may be lacking underscores the importance of making data collection efforts count as much as possible. As mentioned earlier, cardiac arrest data can be used for direct evaluation of cardiac arrest care, for evaluation of successful performance of certain skills, on both a system and a personal level, and for strategic planning.

Summary

Evaluation of the treatment of cardiac arrest resulting from cardiovascular disease is the best tracer available today for EMS system QA. This evaluation can also be used to evaluate the overall care of cardiac arrest victims and to assess system performance, integration of system components, and individual performance of critical parameters. QA of cardiac arrests should not preclude evaluation of other conditions treated by the EMS system, but should instead serve as the cornerstone for all of the system's QA.

REFERENCES

1. Becker LB, et al: Outcome of CPR in a large metropolitan area—Where are the survivors? *Ann Emerg Med* 20(4):355-361, 1991.
2. Bergner L et al: *Evaluation of paramedic services for cardiac arrest.* In: *National Center for Health Services research report series,* DHHS Publication No. (PHS) 82-3310, Washington, D.C., 1981.
3. Cayten CG: *Evaluation of emergency medical services systems.* In: *EMS medical directors handbook,* St. Louis, 1989, Mosby—Year Book.
4. Cobb LA, Alaveraz H III, Copass MK: A rapid response system for out-of-hospital cardiac emergencies, *Med Clin North Am* 60:283-290, 1976.
5. Cummins RO et al: Recommended guidelines for uniform reporting of data from out-of-hospital cardiac arrest: the Ustein style, *Ann Emerg Med* 20:861-874, 1991.
6. Donabedian A: The quality of care: how can it be assessed? *JAMA* 260(12):1743-1748, 1988.
7. Drake L, Thompson M: *Systems design in human resources in prehospital care.* In Cleary VL, editor: *Administrative and clinical management,* Rockville, Md, 1987, Aspen Publications.
8. Eisenberg MS: *Quality assurance: is it possible?,* EMS Forum, ACEP Scientific Assembly, San Francisco, Nov. 1987.
9. Eisenberg MS, Bergner L, Hearne T: Out of hospital cardiac arrest: a review of major studies and a proposed uniform reporting system, *Am J Public Health* 70:236-240, 1980.
10. Eisenberg MS, Horwood BT, Cummins RO: Cardiac arrest and resuscitation: a tale of 29 cities, *Ann Emerg Med* 19:179-186, 1990.
11. Eisenberg MS et al: Survival rates from out-of-hospital cardiac arrest: recommendations for uniform definitions and data to report, *Ann Emerg Med* 19:1249-1259, 1990.
12. Kessner DM, Kalk CE, James S: Assessing health quality—the case for tracers, *N Engl J Med* 288:189-194, 1973.
13. Maio RF: Unpublished data, 1991.
14. Maio RF, Burney RE: Improving reliability of abstracted prehospital care data: use of decision rules, *Prehosp Disast Med* 6(1):15-20, 1991.
15. Pantridge JF, Geddes JS: A mobile intensive care unit in the management of myocardial infarction, *Lancet* 2:271-273, 1967.
16. Polnitsky CA et al: Prehospital coronary care: proposal for a uniformed reporting system, *JAMA* 237:134-139, 1977.
17. Ryan J: *Quality assurance.* In *EMS medical directors handbook,* St. Louis, 1989, Mosby—Year Book.
18. Stout JL: Measuring response time performance, *J Emerg Med Serv* 12(9):106-11, 1987.
19. Stout JL: Measuring your system, *J Emerg Med Serv* 8(1):84-91, 1983.
20. Valenzuela TD et al: Cost-effectiveness analysis of paramedic emergency medical services in the treatment of prehospital cardiopulmonary arrest, *Ann Emerg Med* 19:1407-1411, 1990.

Appendix

Tools for Quality Improvement

Robert A. Swor, D.O.
Ronald G. Pirrallo, M.D.

An important component of any quality improvement (QI) program is the use of tools to identify issues and to assess the impact of changes. The research methods discussed previously in the text are one means by which analysis can be done and hypotheses can be tested. Yet a number of other tools are also useful and relatively easy to apply. They are widely applied in many industries to clarify issues and to suggest solutions.

Analysis is one area in which technical support, in the form of statisticians or industrial engineers, is of value. Many emergency medical services (EMS) systems with affiliations with large hospitals and universities have access to these support personnel. For all but the most basic of evaluations, consultation should be obtained prior to the initiation of data collection. This ensures that adequate data are collected in the appropriate format and that the appropriate method is used.

This overview of additional QI tools is, by necessity, cursory. Readers are referred to a number of excellent reviews (Plsek,[4] Scholtes,[5] and others) for a more complete discussion of the topic.

Microcomputers

The evolution of microcomputers has had a remarkable impact on the ability to collect, analyze, and display data. Both Apple- and IBM-based systems and commercial software are readily available and affordable for this task. For virtually all but the largest EMS systems, hardware can be purchased for less than $5000. Software that supports the user's needs must be obtained. Data

240

management programs (e.g., Dbase IV, Foxpro, and Paradox) are used to collect and to report data and can handle large volumes of data (up to 100,000 records). Spreadsheet programs (e.g., Lotus 1-2-3, Excel, and Quattro) have fairly sophisticated statistical and graphic functions, which can be used to perform data analysis and produce graphic displays.

Flow Diagrams

Flow diagrams effectively clarify the steps of a process and facilitate the understanding of that process. Their major value is to allow personnel to describe a process and identify critical steps that may improve the process. The construction of a flow diagram should include personnel from each step in the process, all of whom should give detailed information as to how the process actually works. Similarly, a flow diagram can be used to test a problem's hypothesized solution before it is implemented.

Cause-and-Effect Diagrams

Cause-and-effect diagrams, first introduced in Japan by Dr. Kaoru Ishikawa, have been referred to as "fishbone," or "Ishikawa," diagrams. They are used to identify and display theories about the causes of a problem. They are most productive when used by teams because they allow personnel from different areas to consider theories from another's perspective. Also, by identifying all possible theories to explain a problem, they identify which data must be collected to evaluate the theories.

Pareto Analysis

Pareto analysis diagrams are used to identify and rank the factors that are the major contributors to a given effect. Two steps are required: the collection of data on factors contributing to a given problem and the graphical display of this data. The underlying theory behind this method is that "whenever a number of individual factors contribute to some overall effect, relatively few of those items account for the bulk of the effect."[2] Identifying and quantifying problems should allow identification of the flaws that contribute most to a problem and that, when corrected, yield the most benefit. See Figure 7-2 on page 78 of Chapter 7 for an example of a Pareto analysis.

Opinion-based Tools

Opinion-based tools are used to generate hypotheses regarding a given process or event but do not generate data to document the validity of a hypothesis. They are a method of assessing perceptions of a given problem. Although valuable techniques to initiate an analysis, they cannot be substituted for data collection.

Delphi and other techniques test perceptions of possible causes of a given problem. Such techniques are performed in an anonymous fashion to collect the individual opinions of the group members. The collated opinions are then returned to the original group to assess the responses.

The nominal group process collects opinions from a variety of individuals without critical comments. It then allows members of the group to discuss opinions generated by individuals in the group.

Similarly, brainstorming sessions allow individuals to generate opinions on a given problem, which are then used to develop possible solutions. Typically these are performed without discussion of each idea to prevent members from fearing judgment and being discouraged from voicing their opinions.

Again, all of these methods are effective for identifying issues but do not generate data.

Graphic Displays

Graphics are invaluable in illustrating and documenting a process. They are the "pictures worth a thousand words" when used to facilitate the review of a process. Patterns of data may be identified, outliers noted, and frequency of problems visualized. Common methods used include the following:

- *Histogram frequency distribution charts* to display variation of continuous data.
- *Line, bar, and pie graphs* to compare frequency and distributions of data.
- *Scatter diagrams* to illustrate the relationship between two given characteristics.

Graphics are a basic component of all major spreadsheet packages, and graphs are relatively easy to create with these programs.

Descriptive Statistics

Methods are needed for summarizing or describing measurements of groups or populations. For categoric data, rates or proportions are often used and are defined as follows:

- A *rate, or proportion,* is defined as being the number of individuals in the category of interest divided by the total number of individuals in the group. The individuals counted in the numerator must be members of the group represented by the denominator.
- The *incident rate* is the proportion of any fixed group developing an attribute or event within a specified time period. Incidence is thus a measure of frequency over time and should always be expressed as a function of time.

STEPS IN PROBLEM SOLVING		QUALITY IMPROVEMENT TOOLS									
		Flow Diagrams	Brainstorming	Cause-Effect Diagrams	Data Collection	Graphs and Charts	Stratification	Pareto Analysis	Histograms	Scatter Diagrams	Control Charts
Defining the Problem	1. List and prioritize problems	○	○		●	○	○	●			
	2. Define project and team	○				○	○				
The Diagnostic Journey	3. Analyze symptoms	●			●	○	○	●	○		○
	4. Formulate theories of causes	○	●	●			○				
	5. Test theories	●			●	●	●	●	●	●	●
	6. Identify root causes	●			●	●	●	●	●	●	●
The Remedial Journey	7. Consider alternative solutions	●	●	○			○				
	8. Design solutions and contols	●			●	●	○		○	●	●
	9. Address resistance to change	○	●	○							
	10. Implement solutions and controls	●				○		○	○	○	
Holding the Gains	11. Check performance	○			●	●	●	●	●	○	●
	12. Monitor control systems	○			●	●	●		○		●

Legend: ● Primary or frequent application of tool; ○ Secondary, infrequent, or circumstantial; ☐ None or very rare

Figure A-1
Applications for QI tools. (From Berwick DM, Godfrey AB, Roessner J: *Curing health care*, San Francisco, 1990, Jossey-Bass Inc.)

A measure of central tendency is a measure that locates the center of the distribution of continuous data. The three most common and useful measures are defined as follows:

- The *arithmetic mean* of a set of *n* measurements is equal to the sum of the measurements divided by *n*. This is often referred to as the average and is sensitive to extreme values.
- The *median* is the actual value of the measurement that falls in the middle when the measurements are ranked in order from the smallest to the largest. The median is less sensitive to extreme values.
- The *mode* is the measurement that occurs most frequently. If all the measurements are unique, the mode does not exist.

Control Charts

Control charts are used to identify and illustrate variations in a process. Using statistical methodology, control limits are calculated based on the range of variation of the data. The calculation is complex and based on work done by Juran[2] and others. This method can be used to identify outliers that need further review. (See Chapter 6 for an example.) These charts are also valuable when monitoring a process once changes have been instituted.

Summary

The reader can use a variety of methods to describe and assess a process, most of which can be applied in an expeditious fashion. The table from Plsek[4] (see Figure A-1) suggests the most effective application of these and other methods for diagnosing and for correcting problems.

REFERENCES

1. Dawson-Saunders B, Trapp RG: *Basic and clinical biostatistics*, East Norwalk, Conn, 1990, Appleton-Lange Publishers.
2. Juran JM: *Juran's quality control handbook*, New York, 1988, McGraw-Hill.
3. Klein KA: *Data collection, analysis, recommendations and evaluation*. In: *Quality assurance in air medical transport*, Orem, Utah, 1990, WordPerfect Publishing Co.
4. Plsek PE: *A primer on quality improvement tools*. In *Berwick DM et al: Curing health care*, San Francisco, 1990, Jossey-Bass Publishers.
5. Scholtes PR: *The team handbook*, Madison, Wis, 1991, Joiner Associates.
6. Spath PL: *Innovations in health care quality measurement*, 1989, American Hospital Assoc Publishing.

Index

Other Mosby Texts of Interest

BOOK CODE	AUTHOR/TITLE	PUBLICATION DATE
01472	Emergidose Slideguides: Pocket Pediatric/Neonatal Emergency Drugs Guide, 2/e	8/91
01471	Emergidose Slideguides: Binder Pediatric/Neonatal Emergency Drugs, 2/e	7/91
06157	Emergidose Slideguides: Pocket IV Anesthetic/Muscle Relaxants/Shock Management	1/87
06161	Emergidose Slideguides: Binder IV Anesthetic/Muscle Relaxants/Shock Management	
06158	Emergidose Slideguides: Pocket Toxicologic Emergencies	1/87
06162	Emergidose Slideguides: Binder Toxicologic Emergencies	1/87
01969	Gonsoulin: Prehospital Drug Therapy	10/93
01932	Gosselin-Smith: Mosby's First Responder Workbook, 2/e	10/88
01751	Grauer: ACLS: Certification Preparation and a Comprehensive Review	8/87
02937	Grauer: ACLS: Mega Code Review Study Cards	7/88
00174	Grauer: ACLS: Instructor's Kit	12/89
02002	Grauer: ECG Interpretation Pocket Reference	9/91
02159	Grauer: Practical Guide to ECG Interpretation	9/91
02927	Huszar: Early Defibrillation	6/91
02410	Huszar: Basic Dysrhythmia Interpretation and Management	7/88
07203	Huszar: Basic Dysrhythmias, 2/e	6/93
03353	Judd: First Responder: Textbook/Workbook Package, 2/e	10/88
06195	Krebs: When Violence Erupts	4/90
05854	Kuehl: National Association of EMS Physicians EMS Medical Director's Handbook	8/89

BOOK CODE	AUTHOR/TITLE	PUBLICATION DATE
06580	Kuehl: National Association of EMS Physicians EMS Medical Director's Handbook, 2/e	9/93
06138	Lee: Flight Nursing: Principles and Practice	9/90
06295	London: Color Atlas of Diagnosis After Recent Injury	2/91
05853	Mack: EMT Certification Preparation	2/90
03375	Madigan: Prehospital Emergency Drugs	3/90
05791	Miller: Manual of Prehospital Emergency Medicine	3/92
03351	Moore: Vehicle Rescue and Extrication	9/90
03227	Mosby's Medical and Nursing Dictionary, 3/e	11/89
04267	Parcel: Basic Emergency Care of the Sick and Injured, 4/e	12/89
04303	Rosen: Emergency Medicine: Concepts and Clinical Practice, 3/e	4/92
05315	Rosen: Essentials of Emergency Medicine	11/90
04284	Rothenberg: Advanced Medical Life Support	11/87
00443	Seidel: Mosby's Guide to Physical Examination, 3/e	12/90
04894	Simon: Pediatric Life Support	11/88
06404	Thibodeau: Structure and Function, 9/e	10/91
05067	Touloukian: Pediatric Trauma	10/90
05321	Ward: Prehospital Treatment Protocols	3/89
03525	Yvorra: Mosby's Emergency Dictionary	10/88
06579	NAEMSP: Quality Management in Prehospital Care	1/93

FOR ORDERING INFORMATION, CALL 1-800-426-4545.